"Laura Harris Smith has proven ██████████████
have peace, rest, energy and clarity when you are naturally
supernatural!"

Sid Roth, host, It's Supernatural!

"Laura Harris Smith has never shied away from telling it like it is, and if you want both spiritual and practical input into the problems you face, you want to grab *The Healthy Living Handbook*. It's accessible, it's bite-size and it'll change the way you view—and live—your own life!"

Steve Best, producer/host, United Christian Broadcasters
of the United Kingdom

"As a Christian physician, I have enjoyed Pastor Laura's *Healthy Living Handbook* tremendously! She offers well-balanced insights into who each of us is: spirit, mind and body. Scripturally based throughout, this handbook offers practical suggestions about how we can cooperate with our heavenly Father as He transforms our lives."

Kenneth C. Parsons, M.D.

"Laura shares profound insight and wisdom that lead to true health and shalom, the life of abundance God intends for all of us as His beloved kids. This is a comprehensive, practical guide that challenges and empowers anyone willing to embrace a lifestyle that catapults them from surviving to thriving."

Tamara Rowe, The Wellness Coach

"Laura challenges and inspires yet again with a practical and attainable formula for spirit-filled living and a healthier existence."

Debra Fraser, president and CEO, Total Living International

"With a pastor's heart and a nutritionist's expertise, Laura Harris Smith has created a road map for enjoying the natural as well as the supernatural benefits of making your health a priority. I have a much greater appreciation for how God designed the 'trinity' of spirit, mind and body to work together for our good—and His glory—after having read *The Healthy Living Handbook!*"

Roger Marsh, staff announcer, FOX Broadcasting

"*The Healthy Living Handbook* shares some very doable ways to gain a healthier spirit, mind and body. Laura's expertise will have you feeling like an expert as well."

Jean Driscoll, eight-time Boston Marathon champion; U.S. Olympic Hall of Fame athlete

"The 'gutsy guidance' Laura Harris Smith gives readers in *The Healthy Living Handbook* combines the straight talk of a pastor's wife, the wisdom of a trusted friend and the sound counsel of a certified nutritionist to help you to achieve a stronger, sounder and God-glorifying body, mind and spirit!"

Rabbi Jonathan Bernis, president and CEO, Jewish Voice Ministries International

"*The Healthy Living Handbook* is absolutely superb. It is both inspirational and informational, with very practical, love-filled and prayerfully rich summations at the end of each chapter to help a broad spectrum of audiences. A must-read for anyone looking to enrich his or her whole being—body, mind and spirit. What a blessing!"

Elisa Sharps, N.D., executive director, International Institute of Original Medicine

THE
HEALTHY
LIVING
HANDBOOK

THE
HEALTHY
LIVING
HANDBOOK

SIMPLE, EVERYDAY HABITS
FOR YOUR BODY, MIND AND SPIRIT

LAURA HARRIS SMITH,
C.N.C., B.S.O.M.

Chosen
a division of Baker Publishing Group
Minneapolis, Minnesota

Published by Chosen Books
11400 Hampshire Avenue South
Bloomington, Minnesota 55438
www.chosenbooks.com

Chosen Books is a division of
Baker Publishing Group, Grand Rapids, Michigan

Printed in the United States of America

Library of Congress Cataloging-in-Publication Data is on file at the Library of Congress, Washington, DC.

ISBN 978-0-8007-9788-1

Unless otherwise indicated, Scripture quotations are from The Holy Bible, English Standard Version® (ESV®), copyright © 2001 by Crossway, a publishing ministry of Good News Publishers. Used by permission. All rights reserved. ESV Text Edition: 2011

Scripture quotations identified BSB are from The Holy Bible, Berean Study Bible, BSB. Copyright ©2016 by Bible Hub. Used by Permission. All Rights Reserved Worldwide.

Scripture quotations identified EASY taken from the HOLY BIBLE: EASY-TO-READ VERSION © 2014 by Bible League International. Used by permission.

Scripture quotations identified ERV are from the English Revised Version.

Scripture quotations identified HCSB are from the Holman Christian Standard Bible®, copyright © 1999, 2000, 2002, 2003, 2009 by Holman Bible Publishers. Used by permission by Holman Bible Publishers, Nashville, Tennessee. All rights reserved.

Scripture quotations identified ISV are from Scripture taken from the Holy Bible: International Standard Version®. Copyright © 1996–forever by The ISV Foundation. All rights reserved internationally. Used by permission.

Scripture quotations identified NASB are from the New American Standard Bible®, copyright © 1960, 1962, 1963, 1968, 1971, 1972, 1973, 1975, 1977, 1995 by The Lockman Foundation. Used by permission. (www.Lockman.org)

Scripture quotations identified NIV taken from the HOLY BIBLE, NEW INTERNATIONAL VERSION®. Copyright © 1973, 1978, 1984 Biblica. Used by permission of Zondervan. All rights reserved.

Scripture quotations identified NIV2011 are from the Holy Bible, New International Version®. NIV®. Copyright © 1973, 1978, 1984, 2011 by Biblica, Inc.™ Used by permission of Zondervan. All rights reserved worldwide. www.zondervan.com

Scripture quotations identified NKJV are from the New King James Version®. Copyright © 1982 by Thomas Nelson, Inc. Used by permission. All rights reserved.

Scripture quotations identified NLT are from the Holy Bible, New Living Translation, copyright © 1996, 2004, 2015 by Tyndale House Foundation. Used by permission of Tyndale House Publishers, Inc., Carol Stream, Illinois 60188. All rights reserved.

Quiet Brain® is a registered trademark of Laura Harris Smith.

Cover design by LOOK Design Studio

17 18 19 20 21 22 23   7 6 5 4 3 2 1

For Trish, who has mentored me in nutrition for the last two decades, who inspired me to eat what I thought was inedible and love it, who shared with me the latest and greatest miracle minerals and who, most of all, carried my heaviest burdens in privy prayer. Thank you for our sisterhood, Queen Trish, and, when I was fighting for my life, for introducing me to . . .

Elizabeth: Thank you for teaching me that food is indeed medicine and for being the first health professional I knew who was interested in the story of my whole body, mind and spirit. Bless you for every email, handout and discount. Not only would I not be alive without you, but the tens of thousands who have now come to me for help might not be, either.

Ladies, you sowed your seed into the right soil. Behold your bounty!

CONTENTS

INTRO

As Easy as One, Two, Three

If you had a dollar for every time you have thought about getting healthier, losing those extra pounds, brightening your aging complexion, eliminating junk foods, better managing your stress, thinking more positively or becoming more spiritually minded, how many dollars would you have accumulated at this point in your life?

Most of us make personal vows regarding our bodies and weight before major holidays because we want to look our best at upcoming events, or even daily when looking in the mirror with dissatisfaction. Countless more of us set new emotional goals every time things get stressful at work or when a draining relationship depletes our joy. As for those new spiritual commitments we make to ourselves and to God, the vast majority of them occur when crisis hits or when everyday prayers feel unanswered. So if you look in the mirror daily, ever encounter stress or feel like a certain prayer is going unanswered, the answer to my question is a staggering dollar amount because it shows that change is constantly on your mind. If you do these just once a day, by the time you are thirty years of age, you will have accumulated $10,950 in well wishes and personal promises. If you are fifty-five, you have racked up $20,075. And if you are seventy, your grand total is $25,550. What if this is the year that you cash in all your chips? What if you actually spend your frequent-desire miles on a makeover?

New Year's seems like the best time to start new and really take ground, but according to University of Scranton research cited in *Forbes* magazine,[1] only 8 percent of us actually keep our New Year's resolutions. So make a New Year's vow if you must, but a new you is available any time of year. What you need for your daily dissatisfactions is a simple daily plan. *The Healthy Living Handbook* is about to change the way you think about getting healthy—body, mind and spirit.

This handbook takes a trinitarian approach to embettering your life, meaning that it divides "you" into the three parts in which God created you, offering healthy living habits for each. Every piece of you gets its very own section, so you can think long and hard about the changes you need to make in that area before moving on. God is three in one, and so are you: You are body, mind and spirit. How can you be sure of this when all you can "see" is your body? You need look no further than the very first chapter of the Bible for the most beautiful proof.

In Genesis 1:26 we already see the Trinity hard at work in the Garden of Eden. God said, "Let Us make man in Our image, according to Our likeness" (NASB). Who are the "Us" and "Our" He is referring to? Whom was God talking to here? None other than the Son and the Holy Spirit. They are three, but one, and so are you. I personally imagine the three of them—still glowing after the ingenious creation of the planets, stars, gravity, mountains, water, clouds, birds, animals, vegetables, minerals

1. Dan Diamond, "Just 8% of People Achieve Their New Year's Resolutions. Here's How They Do It," *Forbes*, January 1, 2013, https://www.forbes.com/sites/dandiamond/2013/01/01/just-8-of-people-achieve-their-new-years-resolutions-heres-how-they-did-it/#3b7ac439596b.

and more—looking down in suspenseful anticipation at the *adamah*,[2] the patch of dirt about to become the Creator's great masterpiece, Adam. I imagine them individually wondering, "What will My part in him look like?" Surely their omniscience did not upstage the wonder of the moment.

Even after God was finished with this masterpiece, just one creature must not have been sufficient to fully embody this amazing three-in-one mystery, and so He also created woman. Genesis 1:27 says, "God created man in His own image, in the image of God He created him; male and female He created *them*" (NASB, emphasis mine). So they are both made by God in His image and together constitute the full "incarnation" of the Trinity's DNA.

These two had a strong desire to love one another, become one flesh and create a third who also embodied the three-in-one Trinity blessing. So beautiful. So mysterious and miraculous. And this beautiful, mysterious, miraculous DNA sprang to life for each of the 108 billion people who have ever been born on this earth.[3] They were all three in one, with body, mind and spirit. It continues today each time God's original design is followed.

And this beautiful, mysterious, miraculous DNA sprang to life for each of the 108 billion people who have ever been born on this earth.

Think you totally understand the Trinity? Here is a good test: Try to explain it to a five-year-old. Five-year-olds will grasp the father and son part, but then try to explain to them how they are not two, but actually one (and remember, most kids that age do not understand Christianese, so you can only use

2. "Lexicon: Strong's H127—'*adamah*," Blue Letter Bible, accessed April 20, 2017, https://www.blueletterbible.org/lang/lexicon/lexicon.cfm?t=kjv&strongs=h127.
3. Carl Haub, "How Many People Have Ever Lived on Earth?," Population Reference Bureau, October 2011, http://www.prb.org/Publications/Articles/2002/HowManyPeopleHaveEverLivedonEarth.aspx.

25-cent words). Once you succeed at that (if you do), throw in the Holy Spirit and see if you can convince the kindergartner that "it" is actually a "He" and that He is one with the Father and Son. Not three, but one—or, even more astonishingly, three *in* one. If you can do this and see the child's eyes light up with revelation, then you truly understand the Trinity in its complex simplicity.

Perhaps it would help to use a practical parable that I have used with my grandchildren: H_2O can manifest as either ice, water or steam. They have three distinct forms: One is solid, one is fluid and one is vapor, but they are all H_2O. Likewise the Father, Son and Holy Spirit are all the same but manifest themselves in different forms. And for that very bright (and skeptical) child who points out it is merely the temperature causing these varied manifestations (H_2O freezes at 32 degrees Fahrenheit and boils at 212 degrees, making steam), you could point out that the Bible indicates there are definite temperature differences in hell and heaven!

If you would rather have a more theological debate with your kindergartner (or yourself), a survey of the New Testament will prove that the "Us" and "Our" from the Genesis account of creation still exist. Numerous Scriptures refer to the Trinity. And its members do not seem to be in a battle for top billing, either. Sometimes the Father is mentioned first and sometimes last. Take a look at the variations in these sequences:

- Spirit, Son, Father (1 Corinthians 12:4–6, John 15:26)
- Spirit, Father, Son (John 14:26)
- Son, Father, Spirit (2 Corinthians 13:14, John 14:16)
- Son, Spirit, Father (Ephesians 2:18)
- Father, Spirit, Son (1 Peter 1:2)
- Father, Son, Spirit (Matthew 28:19 [NKJV], "Go therefore and make disciples of all the nations, baptizing them in

the name of the Father and of the Son and of the Holy Spirit.")

Notice in this Great Commission from Matthew 28 it does not say "in the *names*" of the Father, Son and Holy Spirit, but in the (singular) "name" of them. One name for all three. They are a package deal. Therefore, you cannot come to God without the Son, and you cannot come to Jesus while ignoring His Holy Spirit with whom He wants to invade your life. If you believe in one, you must believe in all. If you disown one, you disown all. And when atheists say there is no God, make no mistake, they are committing the triple sin of also saying there is no Son or Spirit.

The Trinity is a phenomenon even more mind-boggling than the rarity of identical triplets. It defies all mathematical logic, because it does not "add up," figuratively or literally. We naturally gravitate toward easy addition over multiplication, but the mere addition of the Trinity's individual members limits their exponential power when multiplied. They are not $1 + 1 + 1 = 3$, but $1 \times 1 \times 1 = 1$.

> The Trinity is a phenomenon even greater than the rarity of identical triplets. It defies all mathematical logic. They are not $1 + 1 + 1 = 3$, but $1 \times 1 \times 1 = 1$.

So for the five-year-old (or fifty-year-old) who can truly fathom this three-in-one concept of the Trinity, another revelation has instantly been granted him or her: the comprehension of the miraculous design of mankind as a lesser trinity, a three-in-one creature, made in the image of the Father, Son and Holy Spirit. To genuinely understand one trinity is to understand both. But just as I am amazed at how people walk through this world without understanding the delicate triune relationship between the Father, Son and Holy Spirit, I am equally stunned at how many people walk with *themselves* day in and day out and have no clue that they are also made of three parts. How can one ignore his own spirit? And yet, he does. How can one disregard her own emotions? It happens all the time. And how can we pay no attention to our own bodies? This is what we do whenever we ignore a symptom or some other clue that our bodies are crying out for change, or even when we sin with our bodies. We treat ourselves as less than the multilayered miracle that we are.

Likewise, when something goes physically wrong and a diagnosis comes, we often only treat one-third of ourselves. We fill a prescription for our bodies but never address the mind and spirit to learn the disease's origin. Look at that word again: *dis-ease*. When we are not at ease in our minds or spirits, disease often follows in our bodies. Disease is sometimes caused by a "dis-ease." Not that everything in life comes with perfect "ease," but we can walk through the not-so-easy seasons of life with great peace if we truly know the Prince of Peace.

If you do not have peace in your mind, you will not have peace in your body. If you do not have peace in your spirit, you will not have peace of mind. It is the same concept behind what was previously stated: If you disown one member of the Trinity, you disown them all. You cannot segregate the Father, Son and Holy Spirit, and likewise you cannot segregate your body, your mind and your spirit. Not if you want to be whole.

This book will begin with your spirit . . . because! A spiritual foundation is necessary for the rest of the book to bear lasting fruit in your life. There you will get a taste of what it would be like to have me shepherd or "pastor" you. If you were an actual member of the church that my husband and I pastor in Nashville, Tennessee—an interdenominational church we planted in 2004 called Eastgate Creative Christian Fellowship— this shepherding might happen in the hallways or at a church meeting or in a phone call. If you actually attended Eastgate, I would guard over your spirit and encourage you to grow. I would challenge you toward change and ask God to give you a "holy dissatisfaction" if He sees you are settling for anything less than a clean bill of spiritual health. Ask anyone who goes to Eastgate and he or she will tell you that, as a church, we do not let any grass grow under our spirit feet. We are always reaching and growing and evaluating and accomplishing. As we often say, if you do not want to be free, do not come to Eastgate. As such, to the best of my abilities, I want to offer you that same freedom within the pages of this book.

Section 1, for your spirit, will start with a jolt, may occasionally step on your toes and will confront anything in you that prevents spiritual growth. You will either love me or leave me by the end of it, but I think you will love me (plus the challenges) and stick around 'til the end. The healthy living habits there are meaty and provocative, meaning they are intended to provoke you to action. The bold advice and gutsy guidance in Section 1 has long proven to resonate with those I have pastored and parented and has borne good fruit for many. Mind you, it will come minus the accountability, hugs and shoulder to cry on, but until you come to Eastgate for a visit so that I can actually pray for you (or stick around for good so we can mentor you), it will have to suffice. I want to help you be your best you yet.

Some of the healthy living habits are longer than others because some are more complex than others (e.g., it takes fewer words to convince someone to eat his vegetables than it does to get him to forgive the person who broke his heart). For this reason, Section 1—on your spirit—is a little longer overall. And even though the advice in it is not meant to replace your pastor's counsel, as I said, it will be very pastoral in nature because I love sheep (white, black and shorn) and am a shepherdess at heart.

Then, in Section 2, for your mind, I shift from pastor to counselor and teacher, pulling from my decades of experience as both. There I will be an honest friend to you (you have my word). Finally, in Section 3, for your body, I will put to use my certification as a nutritionist and my degree in original medicine to become your nutritionist! Be smart with this advice, but do not let it replace the counsel of your personal nutritionist or doctor; rather incorporate it with their blessing, explaining to them that you are pursuing a body, mind and spirit makeover. Each of your three parts has its own real estate in this handbook so that you can focus on them one at a time and then incorporate them in your day-to-day life.

Many of you have read my last book, *The 30-Day Faith Detox: Renew Your Mind, Cleanse Your Body, Heal Your Spirit* (Chosen Books, 2016), and completed the thirty-day challenge. You lost weight (one man in Tennessee lost 49 pounds in thirty days), brightened your skin and found your hip bones and cheekbones again. A great number of you were even able to lay down your medications afterward for ailments like diabetes, high blood pressure, depression, allergies and more, under your doctors' supervision. The results that poured in from all over the world surprised even me. Countless numbers of you experienced healing in your relationships—with parents, children, difficult friendships, marriages—and thousands more released emotions of bitterness, grief, anger, fear, etc., and found joy and faith again. You wrote me from continents near and far asking for help for your next step in keeping your body, mind and spirit healthy for good this time. Well, this book is the answer to that request. Many of you goal setters are going to treat this book like another thirty-day challenge and focus on incorporating one of the thirty simple habits at a time into your everyday life. You will spend ten days on your spirit in Section 1, ten days on your mind in Section 2 and ten days on your body in Section 3.

> Many of you goal setters are going to treat this book like another thirty-day challenge and focus on incorporating one of the thirty simple habits at a time into your everyday life.

Others of you are going to consume the information like you are cramming for a test, then leave the book on your nightstand to stare you down and challenge you toward a lifestyle of wholeness each new day. Whichever describes the way you read this book, afterward you will be the healthiest version of yourself ever! Are you ready to cash in your frequent-desire miles and wishing dollars and get to work? It is as easy as one, two, three, so let's start with number one: your spirit.

The Top 10
Healthy Living Habits
for Your *Spirit*

1

Be Naturally Supernatural

Something in you longs for the supernatural because a supernatural God created you. You will never be content with your life if it is devoid of supernatural activity—or if you dismiss its authenticity, period. You will never fully look like Jesus, as you are praying to do, if you do not include the supernatural in your life, for the supernatural was and still is a part of His everyday experience. So what is the "supernatural"? According to *Merriam-Webster's*, it is "departing from what is usual or normal especially so as to appear to transcend the laws of nature." So if you never like to depart from the norm, then you will never experience the supernatural. It transcends the law. It is "above the law."

To be more blunt, the supernatural is a law-breaking blessing. By law a leg should not grow as you hold it, allowing the man you are praying for to stand up straight after living for decades with one leg inches shorter than the other. But it happened to me. That afternoon in 1993, the supernatural broke the laws of nature and, frankly, blew my mind. The man returned to his longtime tailor, who could not figure out why his legs were measuring the same length for the first time since he had known him. Months later, the man invited us to his home—and into his closet—to show off all his new pants with matching leg lengths. He was grinning from ear to ear! I, of course, was crying.

The next time the supernatural broke the law in my world was later that year when I prayed for a man diagnosed with HIV and he was healed, later confirmed by blood work. It was the first time I had been asked to be on the healing prayer team, and the night before I had knelt in my closet to pray, telling God I did not know what to pray or do to get a miracle. I had my faith and the healing Scriptures, but I did not know if I needed to take any steps to activate the supernatural. All I heard God say was, *Heal the lepers.* I told God I did not know any lepers, and I wondered if I was off the hook, since surely no lepers would come to church in the morning. But when the first man in my line told me he had HIV, I *knew* this was the "leper" to whom God referred. So I took a chance. I broke out of my norm. With an authority that came from God's directive to me the night before, my husband and I laid our hands on this man, and the supernatural transcended the laws of nature in his body. He was healed. I had walked with Jesus for seventeen years before experiencing the law-breaking blessing of the supernatural like this, but I have never been the same. That was many miracles ago, but I will never forget those first few because of how they convinced me there was more to Christianity than just receiving grace to live a natural life.

> If you settle for only that which is natural and logical, your life will eventually become dull and unfulfilling.

Because you are made in the image of this supernatural God, if you settle for only that which is natural and logical, your life will eventually become dull and unfulfilling, even though you may not be able to put your finger on why.

24

If you never take risks, you are never using your faith, because faith involves risk. Not irresponsible risk, God-inspired risk. You took a risk when you chose to become a Christian. You take a risk every time you choose to give someone the fifty dollars you are going to need next week. I guess you could say I even took a risk by laying my hands on a man with HIV because in the early nineties people still had a lot of fear that they could catch HIV by just being near someone. It is reputationally risky every time you choose to test God's power and ask people if you can pray over them. The supernatural is not "safe" to your flesh, but your spirit is right at home with it. If you would rather live a comfortable, predictable life that excludes risk and faith, you will never tap in to the supernatural side of God. If, on the other hand, you want to believe (and behave) in the supernatural but are not sure how to get rid of your flesh that prefers its comfort zone, I find that it only takes one good total food fast. You must decrease so He can increase (John 3:30), and fasting accomplishes this. I will say more about that in our Top 10 list for the body, under number 9, "Live Life in the Fast Lane."

There is never a dull moment with the supernatural. The Holy Spirit will whisper things to you like *Your boss needs healing prayer and I need your hands. Are you willing to look foolish so I can draw him to Myself and answer his prayers?* Or He may say, *Do you really want to marry someone who does not share your life values, or can you trust Me to take care of you and lead you to someone who deserves you?* Or maybe, *You were created for more than this hamster wheel you are on. Want to step outside of your comfort zone and find a better life?* God can make the supernatural manifest itself in many different ways in your life, but the key is to learn what it is (and what it is not) so that you never miss it—Him—when He calls your name.

Sid Roth is the creator and host of *It's Supernatural!*, a show that focuses entirely on being "naturally supernatural" (his opening quote in each episode) in everyday life. He goes into 2.2 billion homes around the planet on various secular and Christian networks. Sid and his staff have invited me on twice, once with my book on dreams, *Seeing the Voice of God: What God Is Telling You through Dreams and Visions* (Chosen Books, 2014), and once for *The 30-Day Faith Detox*. Both times I was blown away by my experience.

Turns out this wildly popular anchor desk–guest interview show, which soundly educates billions of people about the supernatural, is just the outside wrapper for Sid's amazing ministry, called Messianic Vision. Sid is a Jewish believer in Yeshua and funnels much of the proceeds from *It's Supernatural!* back into Israel and the ministry he has established there to accomplish the great end-time harvest of Jews (Romans 11:26, "All Israel will be saved"). He holds rallies in Israel and the Jews come to Jesus—by the thousands, they come to Jesus—*because of the supernatural*. With his gentle and meek demeanor, Sid, now in his late seventies, takes the stage and asks those who need physical healing to stand, and he prays one prayer for them all. He takes a faith risk, as I described before, knowing that God will back him up, and God always does. Then he asks for a show of hands for those who just experienced a healing change in their bodies, and the hands fly in the air. He then tells them it is Yeshua who has done this for them and invites them forward to receive Him as their Messiah. The thousands of Jews who have been saved through Messianic Vision have done so largely based on an encounter with the supernatural. It is *exactly* the same risk-taking miracle ministry Jesus had when He was on this earth—employing the supernatural to transcend the laws of nature as a means of fostering faith. This is evidenced in John 10:38 (NLT), when Jesus says, "But if I do his work, believe in the evidence of the miraculous works I have done, even if you don't believe me. Then you will know and understand that the Father is in me, and I am in the Father." In other words, "If you don't believe in Me, at least believe the miracles! Then you will understand who I am and believe it all!"

I have very high regard for Sid as a visionary pioneer who expresses the supernatural in the earth. He does it with humility and uncanny excellence in a day when the supernatural is scoffed at, misused or forsaken. He does it through his show, which educates billions, and through the "treasure inside the wrapper" (Messianic Vision)—and now through the It's Supernatural! Network (ISN), which, in case you are interested in growing in the supernatural in your life, is available *free* on every iPhone, Android phone, iPad, tablet and computer in the world. (Just go to an app store and type *Sid Roth*, then download the ISN app.)

Hence, I knew exactly whom I wanted to survey for this section of *The Healthy Living Handbook*—none other than Mr. Supernatural himself. So I interviewed him. He was gracious enough to answer my two gnawing questions: first, "What is the supernatural's greatest enemy?"

We know *who* its greatest enemy is: Satan. The enemy does not want you to experience the supernatural, because he knows that once you taste it, you will never settle for normal again. But the question was not who, but *what*, and here was Sid's response: "The supernatural's greatest enemy is lack of knowledge and operating by previous bad experience instead of the Word of God."

> The enemy does not want you to experience the supernatural, because he knows that once you taste it, you will never settle for normal again.

I concur with this answer. For years I avoided the supernatural because my opinion of it had soured, both through bad experiences of praying for miracles that did not manifest due to spiritual warfare (which I did not know how to engage in) and through poor media representations of the supernatural. I equated miracles and "miracle workers" with dishonesty and lack of character. How sad, now knowing what I know and having seen the miracles and healings I have! I cannot believe how many years I allowed a few poor representatives of the supernatural to outweigh all the pure ones throughout history and Scripture. Once I resolved my lack of knowledge by learning what the Word of God says about it (versus what others, the enemy or my own experiences shouted at me), my faith was finally able to match the power available to us through our mighty and generous God.

My second question for Sid was, "What is the supernatural's greatest *friend?*"

Again, we know *who* is its best friend: the Holy Spirit. But *what* is its greatest ally? Sid's response was unexpected, and yet I wholeheartedly agreed with it! Conveniently, it was also the topic of our next healthy living habit, "Pray Tell," so I am going to wait and give you Sid's answer there.

Perhaps by now you are asking, "Why begin a health handbook with a lesson in the supernatural?" The short answer is that spiritually healthy people believe in the supernatural. The fuller reason, however, is still very simple: If I can get you to believe in the supernatural and to become a naturally supernatural person, then every other life-changing healthy living habit in this handbook will be a piece of cake for you. You know—a mouthwatering piece of double–chocolate chip cake made with almond flour and stevia dark chocolate.

Healthy Habit Helpers

1. Name one way you are going to bring the supernatural into your workplace and home:

_____

_____

_____

_____

Now put your hand over your heart and pray this aloud with me:

Father God, I want to see more of the supernatural than I currently do in my life. I want to see it at work, at home and everywhere I go. I want to be available to You, O God, to let the supernatural flow through me. I am done with the normal, natural, ordinary life. I want the supernaturally extraordinary life. Right now I trade my life for Yours. My plans for Yours. My temporal mindset for Your eternal one. I welcome the supernatural into my world. Use me to spread it everywhere. In Jesus' name, Amen.

2

Pray Tell

How many books, articles or devotionals have you read about prayer? How many prayers have you actually prayed? How many today? Spiritually healthy people have an instinctual ebb and flow to a thriving prayer life. Look at these definitions of prayer and pick the correct one:

1. a solemn request for help or expression of thanks addressed to God or an object of worship
2. a religious obligation of paying reverence to deity
3. a means of seeking blessing and reminding God of our good works
4. a setting for good confession of mortal sins

If you are thinking, *All of the above*, I beg to differ. While prayer can be a good place for all of those things—requests, thanks, reverence, blessing, confession—none of them define what prayer *is*. I believe that prayer is merely paying attention to God. That simple phrase is my intention, although not my invention.

The first definition above came from the dictionary, the second from a Jewish website, the third from the Pharisee's prayer in Luke 18:12 and the final one from a Catholic website, so they are all legitimate answers. But to limit prayer to activity is to miss the point. What is God doing today? How is He feeling at present? Is He burdened by anything? Pay attention to Him when praying. Refrain from just reading your grocery list of needs. Discern what the Spirit is saying first.

At Eastgate, I often refer to this practice as "listening prayer." But the response I get 75 percent of the time when it hits new ears is, "I try, but I don't hear anything when I listen!" The person goes on to confess that sitting and listening for what to pray feels like a waste of time because it is so unfruitful, instead of realizing that that "unfruitful mind" is an invitation in and of itself. It is an open door, not a dead end. If that "dead end" feeling is your experience, I am here to tell you I have the cure! I do not know of any medical treatment out there that can claim a 100-percent success rate, but I can assure you this practice 100 percent cures "prayer deafness" and "unfruitful mind syndrome." You ready?

It is found in 1 Corinthians 14:15 (KJV). Maybe you have overlooked it your whole life: "What is it then? I will pray with the spirit, and I will pray with the understanding also: I will sing with the spirit, and I will sing with the understanding also."

We have already established in the Intro that you are body, mind and spirit, so it should not be news to you that your spirit is completely separate from your mind. Now apply that distinction to prayer: According to 1 Corinthians 14:14–15, you must have been created with the ability to speak to God using both your mind and your spirit. But what does that look like for each one, and how are they different? The New Living Translation unpacks 1 Corinthians 14:14–15 like this:

For if I pray in tongues, my spirit is praying, but I don't understand what I am saying. Well then, what shall I do? I will pray in the spirit, and I will also pray in words I understand. I will sing in the spirit, and I will also sing in words I understand.

From this one passage (in any translation), Paul gives several clues about what it means to pray with the mind versus with the spirit and why praying in the Spirit is the cure for an unfruitful mind during prayer. Refer back to 1 Corinthians 14:14–15 in both the King James Version and the New Living Translation as you make your way through this list:

1. "Praying in the Spirit" and "praying in tongues" are the same and can be used interchangeably, as Paul does.
2. It is possible to have an unfruitful mind in prayer. (No guilt! It might be the Holy Spirit wooing you to pray in the Spirit.)
3. When we pray in the Spirit (in tongues), we do not understand what we are saying with our minds.
4. Likewise, when we pray in the Spirit (in tongues), we are accomplishing things our "mind prayers" cannot due to our minds' human limitations.
5. Paul seems to acknowledge that this "unfruitful mind" can be a perplexing, common experience, requiring a decision while in prayer: "What am I to do?"
6. It is important to pray both with the spirit and with the mind, as well as to sing in the Spirit and with words we understand.

So there you sit, "paying attention to God" for (1) what to pray and (2) how to pray it to be in full agreement with Him, but you are hearing nothing but crickets. What do you do with this unfruitful silence? Is it a blessing or a curse? It is a blessing, an invitation not to be misspent. Awkward silence in prayer is God making your mind unfruitful because He wants you to employ your spirit instead, working with the Holy Spirit to produce a perfect target-hitting prayer. Let me give you an example:

I once was distraught about a certain couple that left East-gate in our early years. We had walked with their family for years, and, in looking at the situation as objectively as I could, I felt firmly that God did not want them to leave, either. So you can imagine how surprised I was one day while praying fervently for them to come back when the Holy Spirit said to me, *Stop!* I was on a prayer walk and can still take you to the spot on the road where I heard it. My mind had been unfruitful, and yet I had trudged forward in prayer, praying what seemed right in my own eyes, which was for them to return. At the Lord's command to stop, I did. Then

> Awkward silence in prayer is God making your mind unfruitful because He wants you to employ your spirit instead, working with the Holy Spirit to produce a perfect target-hitting prayer.

He said, *Do not pray in the understanding about this again until I release you from praying in the Spirit.* Immediately, the revelation came: God had things to accomplish in them first. My prayers had great faith behind them and would bring them back before they were ready to stay for good. I was getting ahead of God.

Wow. More than a year went by, but I honored God's directive and prayed only in tongues about the situation. At times I felt like I was not praying at all, because, remember, the mind does not understand what the spirit is praying even as the prayer is leaving the lips. But, sure enough, the couple returned, and they came with testimonies of heart changes, which they forthrightly stated had to be completed before they could come back. Oh, were my heart and soul happy! And I have never since doubted the bull's-eye power of praying in the Spirit.

Other times, when we experience the unfruitful mind and begin praying in the Spirit, after a while our minds suddenly become fruitful again and we instantaneously know what the Spirit is directing us to pray. I cannot count the thousands of times this has happened to me in the 25 years since I first began praying in the Spirit. In fact, I have learned to begin my prayer times with praying in the Spirit so that the Lord can make my mind fruitful quicker. I know when to stop using my heavenly language because my mind suddenly becomes supercharged with what to pray, words of knowledge, declarations and prophetic insight. It is like being shot out of a cannon! A revelation of authority comes with it because the Spirit Himself has then told me what to pray! In other words, we *pray* in the Spirit so He can *tell* us what to say—"Pray tell." As I said, it is the cure for "prayer deafness" and "unfruitful mind syndrome."

I can hear someone asking (begging) how they can "learn" to pray in the Spirit, and I am going to address that and other topics in our next healthy living habit, "Let the Spirit Move Ya," since this gift is less about learning and more about receiving. But I sense others are still not convinced that they need this spiritual gift, so I will first address those folks, in whose shoes I once stood.

If you look in chapter 12 of 1 Corinthians—Paul's first letter to the church at Corinth—you will see a list of "gifts" that the Spirit gives to believers (thus the name "spiritual gifts"):

- words of wisdom
- words of knowledge
- faith
- gifts of healing
- the working of miracles
- prophecy
- discerning of spirits

- tongues
- interpretation of tongues

I have never met anyone who refused a present or gift from a loved one, and yet many people refuse gifts from God every day. It never ceases to amaze me how people will make room for the first seven (some more enthusiastically than others) but will draw the line at numbers 8 and 9, speaking in tongues and interpretation of tongues. If that is you, I have a suggestion for resolving this. Ready to hear it?

Start viewing speaking in tongues (and interpretation) as the prayer gift. They are on a gift list, right? Then why look at them like a disability? I mean, you cannot deny them in Scripture, so they have to be reckoned with. And for those who concede that speaking in tongues is in Scripture but believe it belongs exclusively to a dispensation that ended when the apostles died, I would remind you that prayer did not end when the apostles died, nor did the presence of the Holy Spirit, and so neither did the combination of the two: Spirit prayer. I simply cannot imagine the last apostle dying—that would be John—and God saying, "Okay, world! The last apostle is dead, and so, as of today, no more spiritual gifts! And if you had one, you gotta give it back by sundown! No more healings! Enough of faith! No wisdom or prophecy, and, especially, quit using My Holy Spirit to pray!" That would be absurd.

When you view your heavenly language as a gift, and especially when you view it as the prayer gift, it suddenly becomes less intimidating. And the Bible must agree that speaking in tongues is just the simple act of prayer because, remember, Paul called it "praying in the Spirit" in 1 Corinthians 14:14–15 (NLT, emphasis mine): "For if I *pray in tongues*, my spirit is praying, but I don't understand what I am saying. Well then, what shall I do? I will *pray in the spirit,* and I will also pray in words I understand."

Please notice that of the nine spiritual gifts listed in 1 Corinthians 12, the only two that are exclusive to the New Covenant are speaking in tongues and interpretation of tongues. The others were already in the Old Covenant—faith, prophecy, healing, miracles, etc.—but the last two are "new," and by offering them to us I believe God takes the other ancient gifts to a new level. In other words, I find that all of the other spiritual gifts are activated in me when I pray in the Spirit. As I pray in the Spirit, for example, I receive prophecy for someone. As I pray in the Spirit, I get a word of wisdom. As I pray in the Spirit, I increase my faith. This last one, especially, is echoed in Jude 20 (NKJV): "But you, beloved, building yourselves up on your most holy faith, praying in the Holy Spirit . . ."

Remember how I asked Sid Roth in Healthy Living Habit No. 1 what the supernatural's greatest friend is? Here was his answer: "Without a doubt," Sid said, "the supernatural's greatest friend is praying in tongues. The more you pray in tongues, the more power you will have and the more sensitivity you will have to the Holy Spirit." And then he cited several Scriptures, including Jude 20 and Acts 1:8, which we will get to later in this section.

Spiritually healthy people pray, and the healthiest pray in the Spirit.

I hope that you have learned through this healthy living habit that prayer is—at its core— just paying attention to God in listening prayer, and that one of the best ways to accomplish that is by praying in the Spirit. I hope you will see that this is merely the prayer gift, and if you already have it, I pray you use it as a gift and not a gun. I also pray it activates the other dormant spiritual gifts inside of you, starting with your most holy faith. Spiritually healthy people pray, and the healthiest pray in the Spirit.

Healthy Habit Helpers

1. Name one thing that has prevented you from spending the time in prayer that you should, as well as a possible solution:

_____

_____

2. Name one thing that has prevented you from praying in the Spirit (once or forever) and how you would like God to help you with it:

_____

_____

Now put your hand over your heart and pray this aloud with me:

Father God, I know You are three parts, Father, Son and Holy Spirit. Forgive me for ever neglecting any part of You, especially the part that would help me better communicate with You, Your Holy Spirit. Right now I offer up to Him my heart—and my mouth—to do with what You will. In Jesus' name I pray this, Amen.

3

Let the Spirit Move Ya

One of my favorite teachings to bring is on the three ways the Holy Spirit moves in Scripture. The reason is that many people today do not believe that He is still moving or going anywhere, and I love seeing the lightbulbs go off over their heads when they realize what awaits them when they let the Spirit move them. Just as a pond gets stagnant with lack of movement, Spirit stagnancy is a symptom of spiritually unhealthy people. They refuse to be led by His Spirit. He led them to repentance for salvation, and that is enough for them. That is like receiving a criminal pardon and being set free from prison but never stepping foot outside and moving on! We need the river of God's Spirit to carry us wherever it wills and to submit to it with meeked expectancy.

Every time I tackle this topic from a pulpit, I like to start from where we all agree, which is on the various jobs the Bible reveals the Holy Spirit having. So before we look at *how* He moves, let's look at *who* He is and *what* He has done.

Who is the Holy Spirit?

- He is eternal (Hebrews 9:14).
- He is omniscient (John 14:26).
- He is omnipresent (Psalm 139:7).

What does the Holy Spirit do?

- He assisted in creating the world (Genesis 1:2).
- He inspired the writing of Scripture (2 Peter 1:21).
- He convicts us of sin, because He is holy (John 16:8).
- He makes us new when we are born of the Spirit (John 3:5–6).
- He makes His home in our hearts (1 Corinthians 3:16–17).
- He seals all believers at their salvation (Ephesians 1:13–14).

Now we can turn our attention to *how* the Holy Spirit moves. Does He even have any manifestations left after that impressive "what" lineup? Turns out, three Greek New Testament words describe His movements, and through understanding them my seventeen-year relationship with Jesus changed drastically.

The first word is *para*,[1] Greek for "with." *Para* describes how the Holy Spirit draws you toward salvation. John 14:17 (NIV) says, "But you know him, for he lives *with* you and will be in you."

The second Greek word is *en*,[2] meaning exactly what you think: "in." This is when the Holy Spirit moves from merely being with you to living inside you once you are saved. Look at John 14:20 (NIV): "On that day you will realize that I am *in* my Father, and you are *in* me, and I am *in* you." What a movement!

---

1. "Lexicon: Strong's G3844—*para*," Blue Letter Bible, accessed April 20, 2017, https://www.blueletterbible.org/lang/lexicon/lexicon.cfm?t=kjv&strongs=g3844.

2. "Lexicon: Strong's G1722—*en*," Blue Letter Bible, accessed April 20, 2017, https://www.blueletterbible.org/lang/lexicon/lexicon.cfm?Strongs=G1722&t=KJV.

But the third word, *epi*,[3] changed everything for me, and if you have never seen it in Scripture, get ready, because it is going to do the same for you. *Epi* means "upon" and signifies how the Spirit will "come upon" you with power: "But you will receive power when the Holy Spirit comes *upon* you" (Acts 1:8 NLT).

It is this tiny word, *epi*, that has sparked great controversy in the Church for centuries. Whole denominations have broken from one another and new ones have formed over the *epi* theory. Why would it not be good news that the Holy Spirit wants to come upon you with power? But many Christians do not believe it is. I can only tell you that I have never met someone who experienced *epi* who did not believe in it. I am telling you, it exists today as surely as it did in Scripture. God is the same yesterday, today and forever. Once you encounter it, you will never doubt it, but if you have not, you might be tempted to build great arguments against it.

So how does the Holy Spirit move?
- **Para—"with"**
- **En—"in"**
- **Epi-"upon"**

For ten years I lived with the Holy Spirit *para* (with) me, wooing me toward salvation at the age of 10. For seventeen years more I lived with Him *en* me (and still do). But at 27, I first experienced *epi*, which was when the Holy Spirit moved *upon* me in what Scripture calls the "baptism of the Holy Spirit" and I involuntarily spoke in a heavenly language. Later, I will tell you exactly how that happened, but first things first.

Epi is not exclusive to Holy Spirit movement. Other spirits can also try to "come upon" you, and I mean not-so-holy ones (evil spirits). Consider a word you may have seen your whole life: *epi*lepsy. Understand now? An individual is going about his day and suddenly a seizure "comes upon" him and he falls to the ground. And I only call seizures a spirit because Jesus did

---

3. "Lexicon: Strong's G1909—*epi*," Blue Letter Bible, accessed April 20, 2017, https://www.blueletterbible.org/lang/lexicon/lexicon.cfm?t=kjv&strongs=g1909.

in Mark 9:14–29, when He cast out a "deaf and dumb spirit" from the helpless epileptic boy, healing him entirely. I firmly believe no Christian can be possessed of a demon because an evil spirit cannot occupy the same space as the Holy Spirit. But it can "come upon," which explains how Christians can be "under attack." But we are *over*comers!

I grasped this understanding of *epi* because of horrible convulsions I endured for many years, and *epi* is exactly how it felt. I would be standing somewhere and the deaf and dumb spirit would *epi* me, and I would fall to the ground unconscious, unable to hear or speak for hours. This happened more than eighty times until God intervened.

Most people would never ridicule an epileptic falling to the ground and shaking uncontrollably under an evil spirit's *epi*. But let it be the *Holy* Spirit coming upon a person—bringing him to his knees, resulting in shaking or falling to the ground entirely, where God can have his undivided attention—and the person might be much worse than ridiculed. He could be persecuted, called a heretic and utterly rejected. I have experienced it. Strange that some folks are not offended at the enemy's *epi* but are thoroughly disgusted at God's. I cannot help but wonder if ridiculing the Holy Spirit is the on-ramp to the unforgivable sin of blaspheming the Holy Spirit.

The ridicule comes from lack of understanding. When the old me heard the phrases *baptized in the Holy Spirit* or *Spirit-filled*, I bristled. The mere suggestion that I did not have all the Holy Spirit I needed offended me. I *knew* I was Spirit-filled because when the Holy Spirit comes "*en*," He comes all the way in and fills you! So it is incorrect to refer exclusively to charismatic Christians as "Spirit-filled" because, I believe from Scripture, *all* Christians are Spirit-filled. Many, however, have not experienced the Holy Spirit's *epi* and had God's Spirit come upon them, especially with the evidence of speaking in tongues. That is why I believe it all comes down to the *epi* encounter.

But here is the best news: *Epi* is not a onetime experience. We see in the book of Acts that Peter, John and others benefited from it repeatedly, and others around the world still are benefiting every day.

So let's get to what you really want to know (besides my personal story), which is, *Where exactly in Scripture does it say we are supposed to have more than just our original filling of the Holy Spirit at salvation?* We should base everything on God's Word, and that is what it took to convince me that there was more of the Holy Spirit to be had than just Him being "near" or "in" me. Let's start with Jesus' own words to His disciples in John 20:22 (NIV), after His resurrection: "And with that he breathed on them and said, 'Receive the Holy Spirit.'"

So now they had the Holy Spirit, right? Well, yes—but it must not have been "enough," because then He promises them (twice, as He is leaving earth) that more is coming: "And now I will send the Holy Spirit, just as my Father promised. But stay here in the city until the Holy Spirit comes and fills you with power from heaven" (Luke 24:49 NLT).

"Power from heaven"? How and why? He answers those questions the second time He promises more Holy Spirit: "But you will receive power when the Holy Spirit has *come upon* you, and you will be my witnesses in Jerusalem and in all Judea and Samaria, and to the end of the earth" (Acts 1:8, emphasis mine).

So how would they receive power? When the Holy Spirit had come upon (*epi*) them. And why would they need this power? *To be witnesses unto the ends of the earth.* Folks, to reject more of the Holy Spirit is to chop our own legs out from under us in reaching the world for Christ! What if the disciples had refused it? Thank heavens they did not say, "No thanks, Jesus! We already received the Holy Spirit, remember?" I shudder at the thought of how I missed this biblical gift for seventeen years. I hope you will not miss it another day.

Look at these other places in Scripture where the disciples experienced *epi* repeatedly:

- Acts 2:1–13, among themselves: "All of them were filled with the Holy Spirit and began to speak in other tongues" (verse 4 NIV).
- Acts 8:12–19, with the Samaritans: "[They] prayed for them that they might receive the Holy Spirit" (verse 15).
- Acts 9:17, with Paul: "Brother Saul, the Lord—Jesus, who appeared to you on the road as you were coming here—has sent me so that you may see again and be filled with the Holy Spirit" (NIV).
- Acts 10:45–46, with Cornelius: "The gift of the Holy Spirit had been poured out even on the Gentiles. For they heard them speaking in tongues and praising God" (NIV).
- Acts 19:6, with the Ephesians: "When Paul placed his hands on them, the Holy Spirit came on them, and they spoke in tongues and prophesied" (NIV).

As for me, I was a 27-year-old deacon's wife, hungry for something more in God. I did not even know what to call it. But when I saw these Scriptures I asked God for Spirit baptism. I waited for some jarring encounter but felt nothing, and I was not going to fabricate or force my heavenly language. Then, after drifting off to sleep one night, I clearly heard a phrase in a dream—a few syllables in what sounded like another language. My eyes shot wide open and I submitted to the natural urge to repeat the phrase. I wondered if God was baby-stepping me through this the way a father would teach his child her first words. As soon as I said the phrase, though, I immediately repented—I remembered that Paul said in 1 Corinthians 14 that tongues must be interpreted, and I did not have an interpretation! God must have giggled at my self-imposed legalism, but He knew my heart, and so when I prayed 1 Corinthians 14:13 (NKJV), "Let him who speaks in a tongue pray that he may interpret," God gave me an interpretation. And this is exactly what I heard Him say: *Pray for your foot.*

"Really, God? Pray for *my foot*? That's *it*?" It was, to say the least, anticlimactic. But then Psalm 91:11–12 (KJV) came to mind: "For he shall give his angels charge over thee, to keep thee in all thy ways. They shall bear thee up in their hands, lest thou dash thy foot against a stone."

Suddenly I got it. I was praying for my safety! I did not know the words to pray (my mind was unfruitful, as we discussed in "Pray Tell"), so I knew this must be what praying in the Spirit was for. Therefore, I just kept repeating that same little phrase over and over. I was like the lady arriving in a foreign country only knowing one sentence in its language and hoping someone was going to help me find food!

I drifted off to sleep and it happened again. I heard the same exact phrase, then jolted awake. So once again I prayed the phrase, and once again, I prayed for my protection using Psalm 91:11–12. That is all I knew to do. It turned out to be enough.

That very week, with my husband out of town and all our kids in the car with me, I had total brake failure. As I pumped the brake with my foot repeatedly with no result, the prayers for "my foot" flashed through my mind. Before I knew it, I came to a complete stop in the middle of an intersection as if someone had put a hand on top of my car and brought it to a safe stop without my help. I was astonished! It was also a double miracle that no one pummeled us, sitting in the middle of that busy intersection.

> I was like the lady arriving in a foreign country only knowing one sentence in its language and hoping someone was going to help me find food!

Later that week, while on the landline phone, I was struck by lightning traveling through the cord and knocked off my feet. Again, the "foot" prayer flashed through my mind. I was totally safe! This was also during the years when I was having the convulsions—which are basically caused by an overabundance of electricity in the brain—so it is a miracle that it did not throw me into a seizure, or worse.

Those two experiences convinced me I needed this weapon in my prayer arsenal. I employed it immediately, but remember, I only knew this one little phrase. Somehow, I knew God would not reject it, just like I would never reject one of my babies who could only say, "Ma-ma," or, "Da-da," and so I continued on like this for several months.

Then, one night while I was watching Christian television, a pastor gave an altar call for the baptism of the Holy Spirit. I was totally content with praying my potent little phrase of protection over my family (hey, it worked), and so I got on my knees alone in my den and offered it up to the Lord one more time. Then . . . *wham!* Suddenly, as if a river got dumped on top of my head and coursed through my body, the Holy Spirit "came upon" me and began to speak through me fluently in a language I had never learned. I could not stop it or control it. It was even faster than I talk in English, which is pretty fast. Deep calling out to deep, every cell in my body was feeling the reverberation of the call. It was what to this day I refer to as "dish rattling."

All I could do—once it stopped—was worship Jesus. Still on my knees, I fell over on my face, exhausted, and just cried, whispering His holy name over and over. It was as though all at once He had deposited another language in me. Imagine it! The equivalent of, say, not knowing how to speak French and now you can, or not knowing Spanish but now you do. Instantly! I knew I had just been given a full vocabulary that would confound the enemy and commission angels, and to this day I am still using phrases, sentences and words that He deposited in me on that epic *epi* day. The words are still there whenever I summon them, often minus the dish-rattling encounter, but sometimes with. My mind is unfruitful when I use that vocabulary, for I need no other language at that moment in prayer, but as I described in "Pray Tell," before long, my mind is racing with revelation, and I begin to declare and call forth, the result of which is answered prayer. I will never live without this weapon-gift again.

I hope you see from all the cited Scriptures and from my testimony that there is a difference between receiving the Holy Spirit (*en*) upon salvation and being baptized in the Holy Spirit when He comes upon you (*epi*). Did John not prophesy this in Matthew 3:11 at Jesus' baptism? "I indeed baptize you with water unto repentance, but He who is coming after me is mightier than I, whose sandals I am not worthy to carry. He will *baptize you with the Holy Spirit* and fire" (NKJV, emphasis mine).

Also, remember the words Jesus spoke in Matthew 7:9–11 and Luke 11:13, which ends with this: "If you then, though you are evil, know how to give good gifts to your children, how much more will your Father in heaven *give the Holy Spirit to those who ask him*!" (NIV, emphasis mine).

This shows you must ask Him, and I hope I have helped ready you. Whether for the first time or the thousandth, let's ask together now.

Healthy Habit Helpers

1. Name one good reason why you should not receive the baptism of the Holy Spirit:

_____

_____

I hope you could not find one. Now put your hand over your heart and pray this aloud with me:

Holy Spirit, I am ready for more of You. I want all of You there is to be had. Empty me of any doubt You see, and prepare me right now to receive. Fill me, Father. I receive what Scripture calls "power from on high" and the "baptism of the Holy Spirit." I trust You and will wait on You here to move upon me. I love You, Lord! Amen!

4

Get the Word Out

Literally. Get your Bible out and read it more often! It never ceases to amaze me how some people are willing to risk their lives in order to own a copy of the Bible, yet many others have multiple copies lying around their houses and cannot seem to get one read. Spiritually healthy people get the Word out every day.

The Bible was written over a span of 1,500 years by forty different authors (thirty Old Testament and ten New Testament). I had an experience once that forever changed the way I viewed those forty men. I was at a writers' conference, trying to inspire budding authors to pursue their literary dreams. From the small stage I did a quick head count and saw forty writers present. Feeling a surge of temporary genius, I asked them to pretend for a moment that they were the authors of the Bible. Imagine it! All forty biblical authors in the same place! You could feel the inspiration swell in the room because it suddenly humanized the biblical authors and personalized their sacrifices. What if David had considered himself too busy running for his life that he never wrote his psalms? It is one thing to compose and sing a song out loud while you are supposed to be in hiding, but quite another to say, "Whoa! I had better write that one down!" *That* is a song worth reading and even memorizing, because David obviously risked his life for it. What if Ezekiel had dismissed his cryptic visions for pizza dreams and never recorded them, or if Paul had felt sorry for himself in prison and never asked for a papyrus scroll to write his now-famous epistles? And what if Moses had deprioritized recording the Ten Commandments (not to mention that second set of tablets after he smashed the first) and never chronicled Israel's history for us in the book of Exodus?

As an author, I appreciate it when people buy and treasure my writings. I do not want to get to heaven and have Solomon ask me what I thought of his love song and have no answer because I never grasped his intent for penning it. Some biblical authors lost their lives after writing their books. Later, others gave their lives to translate them. Today, many lose their lives trying to transport the Bible or, as I said, just trying to acquire a copy. Surely those of us who have the liberty to possess should exercise the discipline to read.

> Surely those of us who have the liberty to possess should exercise the discipline to read.

Remember Dr. Seuss's *The Cat in the Hat*? More than ten and a half million copies sold to date.[1] What about that red-orange Betty Crocker cookbook that your mother (and probably you) owned? Seventy-five million copies.[2] And I am sure that J. R. R. Tolkien (whose home I once visited in Oxford, England) would be pleased to know that *The Lord of the Rings* and *The Hobbit* together have sold 250 million copies.[3] Take a look at these other bestsellers:

1. Carol Memmott, "After 50 Years, a Tip of the Hat to One Cool 'Cat,'" *USA Today*, February 26, 2007, http://usatoday30.usatoday.com/life/books/news/2007-02-26-cat-in-the-hat_x.htm.

2. Monte Olmsted, "Betty Crocker in Your Kitchen? There's an App for That," *Taste of General Mills* (blog), September 22, 2014, http://www.blog.generalmills.com/2014/09/betty-crocker-in-your-kitchen-theres-an-app-for-that/.

3. Noel L. Griese, "The Bible vs. Mao: A 'Best Guess' of the Top 25 Bestselling Books of All Time," *Publishing Perspectives*, September 7, 2010, http://publishingperspectives.com/2010/09/top-25-bestselling-books-of-all-time/.

- Little House on the Prairie series (Laura Ingalls Wilder), 60 million[4]
- *Catcher in the Rye* (J. D. Salinger), 65 million
- *The Lion, the Witch and the Wardrobe* (C. S. Lewis), 85 million
- *A Tale of Two Cities* (Charles Dickens), 200 million
- The Koran (Muhammad), 800 million[5]

But despite those impressive numbers, the Bible has sold more than all of those books *combined times three* (and maybe more). According to Guinness World Records, the Holy Bible is the bestselling nonfiction book of all time at five billion copies sold.[6] But many think this does not include the two billion copies *given away* by the Gideons, so the number might be closer to seven billion. (It took the Gideons 93 years to distribute the first billion Bibles, but only 14 years for distribution of the second billion.[7] They also report that the Bible is available in 2,426 languages, covering 95 percent of the world's population, and that they give away a Bible every second.[8])

But most powerful of all in these secular statistics is the category that Guinness put the Bible in: nonfiction. This is an acknowledgment that the Bible is entirely true. It is more than just onion-skin paper and ink. It is actually alive! The fact that

---

4. Maria Russo, "Finding America, Both Red and Blue, in the 'Little House' Books," *New York Times*, February 7, 2017, https://www.nytimes.com/2017/02/07/books/review/little-house-laura-ingalls-wilder-anniversary.html?_r=0.

5. Copies printed of the final four titles in this list come from Griese, "Bible vs. Mao," http://publishingperspectives.com/2010/09/top-25-bestselling-books-of-all-time/.

6. "Best Selling Book of Non-Fiction," Guinness World Records, accessed April 20, 2017, http://www.guinnessworldrecords.com/world-records/best-selling-book-of-non-fiction/.

7. "Gideons Distribute Historic Two Billionth Scripture," *The Gideons International* (blog), April 28, 2015, http://blog.gideons.org/2015/04/two-billion/.

8. "The Battle of the Books," *The Economist*, December 19, 2007, http://www.economist.com/node/10311317.

it has far outsold any other book by such broad measures is proof of that life. Although those other literature books are noteworthy, they are dead, as are most of their authors. But the written Word is alive because the Living Word is alive and will live forever: Jesus. "For the word of God is living and active, sharper than any two-edged sword, piercing to the division of soul and of spirit, of joints and of marrow, and discerning the thoughts and intentions of the heart" (Hebrews 4:12).

Unfortunately, the Church teeters on the brink of biblical illiteracy. Beware lest you be counted among them. Many Christians read multiple good books every year but rarely pick up the *best* book of all, the Bible. If you want to get deceived and fall away from your purest faith, do not read your Bible. If you do not want to fall into deception, then you must carve out daily time and be disciplined about studying God's Word.

To help you in this, I want to introduce you to a 1,500-year-old Scripture reading practice called *lectio divina*, which is Latin for "divine reading." In case you are not familiar with it, it involves contemplating a certain area of biblical text—not from a theological or historical standpoint, but with the pure intention of letting the Living Word speak to you concerning it. The four steps of *lectio divina* are to read, reflect, pray and contemplate. Contemplate what? That particular Scripture's application to your life. This type of reading does not treat Scripture as text to be studied or doctrinally dissected, but as the Living Word of God that wants to invade your life at that very moment. You actually view the Scripture with Christ and discuss it with Him. It is a glorious practice, and I cannot wait for you to experience it if you have not.

> The four steps of *lectio divina* are to read, reflect, pray and contemplate.

Get creative with your study of Scriptures. Take, for example, the psalms. Omitting Sundays, there are a little more than three hundred days of the year. So you could spend two days on each of the 150 psalms and practice *lectio divina* with each one, perhaps even memorizing one verse during that two-day period. By the end of the year, you would have memorized 150 Scriptures.

This is too important to miss, so I am going to say it again: If you want to get deceived and fall away from your purest faith, do not read your Bible. If you do not want to fall into deception, then you must carve out daily time and be disciplined about studying God's Word.

Healthy Habit Helpers

1. Name the number-one obstacle that prevents you from reading your Bible daily (e.g., busy schedule, lack of discipline, no desire, etc.):

_____

_____

Now put your hand over your heart and pray this aloud with me:

Father God, I love Your Word, but I want to love it more. I am asking You, right now, to give me an insatiable desire to open it and sit with it and to absorb its every word! God, I give it permission to call out to me, to interrupt what I am doing and to make me miserable if I neglect it. It is alive! I want a living relationship with Your Word! Illuminate Scripture to me as I read, God, and fill me with Your Holy Spirit so I can understand Your truths in full. I ask all of this in Your name, Jesus, Amen.

5

Do the Honors

Pop quiz time. Sorry for the short notice, but you have been studying for this one your whole life. Spiritually healthy people live, sleep and breathe honor. They would rather be physically ill than dishonor those in authority over them. Let's see how well you understand honor.

1. What does the word *honor* mean?
   a. to promote
   b. to honor oneself
   c. to estimate
   d. to fix the value of
   e. all of the above
   f. only *a* and *b*
   g. none of the above

The answer is *e*, all of the above. The Hebrew word for honor is *kabed*,[1] which means many things, including "to promote;

1. "Lexicon: Strong's H3515—*kabed*," Blue Letter Bible, accessed April 20, 2017, https://www.blueletterbible.org/lang/lexicon/lexicon.cfm?t=kjv&strongs=h3515.

to honor oneself." This shows that to honor someone is to give that person a promotion, and that when you give honor, you also honor yourself. In other words, when you use your words or actions to promote someone, you also get promoted! Give honor, get honor. It is the New Testament principle of sowing and reaping.

The Greek word for honor is *timao*,[2] which means "to estimate; fix the value." I *love* this, because it means that when we show someone honor, we are broadcasting to the world the value we have fixed on the relationship and estimated it to be of great worth. When we show respect with our words and actions, onlookers will say, "Wow, look at the honor that person is showing. She obviously put great value on that relationship!" Promotion is in that person's future.

2. Whom will God honor?

   a. those who honor Him

   b. those who serve His Son

   c. those who do good

   d. those in powerful positions

   e. all of the above

   f. only *c* and *d*

   g. *a* through *c* above

The correct answer is *g*, *a* through *c* above. Here are the Scriptures to back that up. God does not automatically honor those in powerful positions, for reasons we will discuss in a moment.

- "For those who honor Me I will honor" (1 Samuel 2:30 NASB).

2. "Lexicon: Strong's G5091—*timaō*," Blue Letter Bible, https://www.blue letterbible.org/lang/lexicon/lexicon.cfm?t=kjv&strongs=g5091.

- "If anyone serves me, the Father will honor him" (John 12:26).
- ". . . but glory and honor and peace to everyone who does good" (Romans 2:10 NASB).

3. What precedes honor?
   a. accepting correction; teachability
   b. obeying your boss
   c. righteousness and loyalty
   d. humility
   e. pride
   f. *a* through *d* above
   g. none of the above

The answer is *f, a* through *d* above, as you can see from these Scriptures:

- "Poverty and disgrace come to those who ignore discipline, but the one who accepts correction will be honored" (Proverbs 13:18 HCSB).
- "Whoever obeys his master will be honored" (Proverbs 27:18 ISV).
- "He who pursues righteousness and loyalty finds life, righteousness and honor" (Proverbs 21:21 NASB).
- "Humility goes before honor" (Proverbs 18:12 NASB; see also Proverbs 15:33).
- "A man's pride will bring him low, but a humble spirit will obtain honor" (Proverbs 29:23 NASB).

4. Whom does the Bible say you should honor?
   a. your parents
   b. gracious women/your elders/church workers

    c. your spouse/marriage/the marriage bed

    d. your government leaders

    e. God and Jesus

    f. others above yourself

    g. all of the above

The answer is g, all of the above, and here are the Scriptures to support those answers:

- "Honor your father and your mother, that your days may be prolonged in the land which the LORD your God gives you" (Exodus 20:12 NASB; see also Ephesians 6:2–3).
- "A gracious woman gets honor" (Proverbs 11:16).
- "The elders who rule well are to be considered worthy of double honor, especially those who work hard at preaching and teaching" (1 Timothy 5:17 NASB).
- "Welcome him in the Lord with great joy, and honor men like him, because he almost died for the work of Christ, risking his life to make up for the help you could not give me" (Philippians 2:29–30 NIV).
- "Marriage should be honored by all, and the marriage bed kept pure, for God will judge the adulterer and all the sexually immoral" (Hebrews 13:4 NIV).
- "Show proper respect to everyone: Love the brotherhood of believers, fear God, honor the king" (1 Peter 2:17 NIV).
- "Be devoted to one another in brotherly love. Honor one another above yourselves" (Romans 12:10 NIV).

So now that you know what *honor* means, whom God honors, what characteristics precede honor in your life and whom to honor, let's talk about who to *not* honor. Society is full of celebrities and public figures who are receiving honor where it is not due. Even some ungodly judges making dangerous decisions for the masses we refer to as "Your Honor." God does not say, "Your Honor," to them or return honor to celebrities who do not meet the above scriptural requirements. If those in powerful positions do not honor their parents, elders, government officials, etc., they will not receive honor themselves. It may temporarily come on earth, but not from God, whether on earth or in heaven. Be careful not to give honor to those who never show it. And by that I mean think twice about whose products you buy, whose movies you see and whose music you listen to. If they are dishonorable in any way, you are sowing into dishonor with your money, time and attention. Read Psalm 12:8 in a couple of different translations:

> The wicked strut about on every side when vileness is exalted among the sons of men. (NASB)

> The wicked wander everywhere, and what is worthless is exalted by the human race. (HCSB)

So, then, the real conundrum comes when you are called upon to honor one who honors none. What do you do with that boss, coach, husband, wife, sergeant, pastor, parent, president or professor who does not honor God or man? Are you still required to honor? Friend, God requires honor of everyone. No one is exempt from it, or the blessings that follow it. But navigating through these tedious relationship land mines takes much prayer and patience. You must pick your battles. So we will discuss that at length under Healthy Living Habit No. 8 for your mind, "Pick Your Battles."

> The real conundrum comes when you are called upon to honor one who honors none.

Begin to notice how you speak to those whom God considers to be in authority over you. Ask Him to give you the language of honor. Southerners teach their children to say, "Yes, ma'am," and, "No, sir," out of honor. If you were standing before the president, you would not call him (or her) by his first name; you would address him as "Mr. President." If you were answering a judge in court, you would not answer his or her questions with "Yeah." You would say, "Yes, Your Honor." You may think the language of honor is purposeless, but I assure you it is not. I will give you a personal example.

When we planted and began pastoring Eastgate, our church was primarily composed of old friends. None of them called us "Pastor" because they had known us for years as "Chris and Laura," and I suppose it felt awkward to tack on a title. Did we care about the title? Actually, not a bit. But in retrospect, it might have helped us to see ourselves in more of a pastoral light. Those early years were tough, as Chris was working two jobs as a bivocational pastor trying to support six kids, and during certain lean seasons, he was trivocational. Then there was me, working several jobs and stoking many professional and creative fires. Eastgate was planted with wonderful apostolic covering but no financial aid, and it was not an easy road. There were times when Chris and I wondered if we were making a difference. We were meeting in a rented space, and to get there we had to pass three prosperous churches with big steeples each week. We did not feel very much like pastors, except for our sheep whom we loved and who loved us. But at home, I would sometimes call Chris "Pastor," because I wanted someone calling him that. I knew it was important. I would call him at his construction job and say, "Hey, Pastor! You are a phenomenal pastor. What other pastor do you know who works three jobs all for the privilege of standing up and ministering to God's people every Sunday? No one but you, Pastor." He would chuckle, but I knew it had an impact.

When the church was about four years old, a new woman came, and after a few months she stood up in the service after someone talked about looking forward to the day when Chris was a full-time pastor. This woman said, "I notice that none of you call our pastors 'Pastor Chris' or 'Pastor Laura.' I also notice that they don't seem to mind. But how is it that we say we want them to be full-time pastors but are not even calling them 'Pastor' full-time? Aren't we supposed to call things that are not as though they are? I am going to call them 'Pastors Chris and Laura,' and you should, too." And she did. Some followed suit and some did not. Some never may, I suppose. But because a base emerged who always referred to us as "Pastor Chris" and "Pastor Laura"—in public, in private, to their children, on the phone, from the pulpit, in the lobby, etc.—new folks who came did, too. And once that happened, sure enough, it was not long before we were full-time pastors. That woman is not even with us any longer, but I honor her for how she honored us. Something shifted in us (and the church) when she challenged everyone. Keep in mind that the language of honor, including the usage of titles, is not meant to puff up your leaders, but to be a constant reminder to them of the weighty responsibility they hold. I can honestly say I have never once spoken disrespectfully to my previous pastors, scowled at them with my facial expressions or gossiped about them behind their backs, not even when I strongly felt they deserved it. I have spoken into their lives, but the truth was spoken in love. I believe some of the honors I am receiving today are a direct result of me showing honor during those hard tests. *Spiritually healthy people crave opportunities to show honor.* I would rather be physically ill than to dishonor a pastor or other spiritual mentor, and I trust I will continue to reap honor from my own congregants as a result.

> The language of honor, including the usage of titles, is not meant to puff up your leaders, but to be a constant reminder to them of the weighty responsibility they hold.

In closing, let's consider some practical ways you can show honor:

1. Honor God by obeying His Word and by ministering to His Body.
2. Salute soldiers or thank them for their service when you see them.
3. Thank law enforcement when you see an officer in public.
4. Honor your teachers by taking care of and rewarding them.
5. Honor your spouse with your words to them and about them.
6. Single out child-care workers at your church and bless them.
7. Bless your boss with your submission and cheerful team-work.
8. Respect your parents with your words, facial expressions and actions.
9. Bless your pastors by being teachable and implementing their counsel.
10. Honor your children by listening to them and teaching them to sow honor everywhere they go so that they might reap it for a lifetime.

Remember that in order to be honored, you must first show honor. Honor is synonymous with promotion, as shown by the Hebrew word we learned earlier: "I thought to promote (*kabed*) thee unto great honour (*kabed*); but, lo, the LORD hath kept thee back from honour (*kabed*)" (Numbers 24:11 KJV).

Promotion and honor are interchangeable! Look at that verse again. Great promotion was withheld. You will never get promoted in life, and you will stay at the same level in your jobs and relationships, unless you learn this secret of honor.

As for the fifth Commandment in Exodus 20:12, how marvelous that God has put promotion in the hands of children. "Honor your parents" becomes "Promote your parents." It is not the other way around. Children do the promoting. And that does not exclude us adult children. "Honor [promote] your father and mother (which is the first commandment with a promise), so that it may be well with you, and that you may live long on the earth" (Ephesians 6:2–3 NASB).

Make a point to study those who honor. They themselves will be honored before long.

Salute

Honor is a way of life, a state of mind, a view
Whether you are showing it or it's been shown to you

It's giving adulation to that teacher in your life
It's listening to your husband or deferring to your wife

It's honoring your parents; a commandment with a vow
That you will live a long and happy life beginning now

It's venerating clergy, taking time to ease their strain
Saluting every soldier; paying homage to the slain

If accolades were silver and respect was bars of gold
We'd stuff our pockets full of both and never dare withhold

But honor isn't just esteem we know we should be giving
It's honest, brave integrity that infiltrates our living

It's holding fast to principles and goodness at all cost
It's guarding reputation so no character is lost

A good name is worth riches and a bad one breaks the bank
So live your life uprightly and it's honor that you'll thank
                                        ©Laura Harris Smith

Outdo one another in showing honor.

Romans 12:10

Healthy Habit Helpers

1. Name the people in your life to whom you know you need to show more honor, and write how you can show it:

_____

_____

_____

_____

Let's pray and ask God to give you a heart to honor. Do not be surprised if He also brings conviction of times when you have been less than honorable with others. Now put your hand over your heart and pray this aloud with me:

Father God, I want to be a person of honor. Forgive me for my lack of it. Show me when I have behaved dishonorably. Give me courage to apologize and change. Help me to understand the link between honor and promotion so that I might be blessed all my days. I ask it all in Jesus' name, Amen.

6

Put On Your Sunday Shoes

Today's title, "Put On Your Sunday Shoes," is a common idiom chosen as a one-size-fits-all (pun intended) for this subject of church attendance, but let me begin by saying that depending on your denomination and church, you may instead own a pair of Friday shoes, Saturday shoes, etc. The aspiration of this commentary is to remind you to wear them weekly. Thirty-seven percent of all Americans attend church weekly, according to a 2013 study by the Pew Research Center.[1] Gallup puts that number at 39 percent.[2]

But ChurchLeaders.com paints a different picture, arguing that less than 20 percent of America is regularly in church.[3] A

---

1. Michael Lipka, "What Surveys Say about Worship Attendance—and Why Some Stay Home," *Fact Tank*, Pew Research Center, September 13, 2013, http://www.pewresearch.org/fact-tank/2013/09/13/what-surveys-say-about-worship-attendance-and-why-some-stay-home/.

2. Frank Newport, "In U.S., Four in 10 Report Attending Church in Last Week," Gallup, December 24, 2013, http://www.gallup.com/poll/166613/four-report-attending-church-last-week.aspx.

3. Kelly Shattuck, "7 Startling Facts: An Up Close Look at Church Attendance in America," *Church Leaders*, December 29, 2015, http://churchleaders.com/pastors/

2015 article states that in the late 1980s, David Olson, director of church planting for the Evangelical Covenant Church, began tracking annual attendance at more than 200,000 Christian churches in America (the accepted U.S. church population is 330,000 congregations[4]). For the other 100,000-plus churches, he used alternative methods like statistical models and membership-to-attendance ratios. This provided a phenomenally accurate representation of almost every church in America—evangelical, Catholic and Protestant.

His thorough study revealed that the accurate measurement of church attendance is less than half of what Gallup, Pew Research Center and other pollsters say: In 2004 only 17.7 percent of Americans went to church on any given weekend. The *Journal for the Scientific Study of Religion* published another study in 2005 by sociologists Penny Long Marler and C. Kirk Hadaway, which backed up Olson's findings, reporting that the actual percentage of people worshiping each week was less than 22 percent, instead of the popular pollster reports of almost 40 percent.[5] Why the discrepancy?

It is called the "halo effect"—a phrase invented by psychologist Edward Thorndike in 1920 to explain why we tend to make judgments about a person's behavior and character based on our overall impression of that person. In this case, people perceived *themselves* as having a "halo" and exaggerated their church attendance. In their study, Marler and Hadaway discovered a clear inconsistency between what people were telling pollsters and what they were really doing.[6] (This proves that people know they need to be in church, which

---

pastor-articles/139575-7-startling-facts-an-up-close-look-at-church-attendance-in-america.html.

4. C. Kirk Hadaway and Penny Long Marler, "How Many Americans Attend Worship Each Week? An Alternative Approach to Measurement," *Journal for the Scientific Study of Religion* 44, no. 3 (2005): 307–322.

5. Ibid.

6. Ibid.

was confirmed by another study stating that on Easter and Christmas, national attendance increases to six out of ten people.[7]) Turns out that in polls, Americans tend to "under-report undesirable behavior like drinking and over-report behavior like church attendance and voting."[8] Even broadening the polling criteria to include Americans who attend three out of every eight Sundays still brings the number only to 23–25 percent.

This should not be so! I am not happy with any percentage under 100 percent, but not because I believe in some sort of legalistic attendance requirement. I believe in 100 percent spiritual health, and 100 percent spiritual health is unachievable when you are dangling off the vine.

I often refer to a church service as the "family table." Everyone brings a dish, helps serve and helps clean up, and your chair is glaringly empty if you are absent. At your family table at home, would you be healthy if you only ate 17 percent of your allotted meals or, when you did eat, only consumed 17 percent healthy foods? No. You cannot skip 83 percent of your meals and consume 83 percent junk when you do eat and expect to *not die* (physically or spiritually). So, if 83 percent of America is not in church regularly, is it any wonder why our nation is in its current state of disrepair, especially the condition of the American family? Friend, you cannot be spiritually healthy unless you are at the family table regularly at your local church. I do not care who you are, how many great devotionals you read (or write), how many charities you support or how many people you lead to Jesus at the gas pump—you are spiritually

7. Ed Stetzer, "What Is Church Attendance Like During Christmastime? New Data from LifeWay Research," *Christianity Today*, December 14, 2015, http://www.christianitytoday.com/edstetzer/2015/december/what-is-church-attendance-like-during-christmastime-new-dat.html.

8. Shattuck, "7 Startling Facts," http://churchleaders.com/pastors/pastor-articles/139575-7-startling-facts-an-up-close-look-at-church-attendance-in-america.html.

malnourished if you are not coming to the family table at least weekly at your local church.

You know, Jesus was a statistician, too. His Parable of the Sower in Mark 4 shows that even with good seed and soil, some crops will yield 30 times what was sown, some 60 times and some 100 times. You see it at your own church. Everybody has access to the same sermon and is living in the region with the same socio-economic influences, and yet people experience various levels of happiness and success. They may not be able to control everything around them, but as for their attitudes and faith levels during trials,

I often refer to a church service as "the family table." Everyone brings a dish, helps serve and helps clean up, and your chair is glaringly empty if you are absent.

their responses vary greatly, even though they all had access to the same message on Sunday about attitude and faith (but all did not go hear it). In farming, this disparity is caused by variations in the elements of agriculture. Did certain people's fields have better access to quality water? Better sunlight? Proper shade? These elements can make all the difference in two crops planted with the exact same seed in the same area's soil. Likewise, the local church is one of the most important variables in providing the proper elements necessary for the field of your life, but you *must* go, plant yourself, let your roots go deep and grow.

So why *do* people deprioritize church if it is so good for them to go? Partial fault lies with churches themselves if they have become dull and irrelevant to society. But the ultimate fault lies with the individual for not searching high and low until he finds a more thriving church. They are out there! Not finding the right church is no excuse for not attending one any more than not finding the right grocery store is an excuse for starving. There are options. This is on you. Put as much energy into finding the right church as you would into finding the right job, and if you are already in a church, put as much effort into getting up and getting there on time as you do getting up and getting to work on time (or more). And show the same amount of effort once you get there.

Now, in case you still do not believe church should be a weekly priority for you, let me ask you these ten questions:

1. Concerning your church leaders (not just the pastor), how can you "imitate their faith" (Hebrews 13:7) if you never or rarely see them?

2. How can you "obey your leaders and submit to them" (verse 17) if you are not attending church and are not well known by its leaders? And how can they "keep watch over your soul" if you are never there?

3. How do you build up the Body of Christ, as Paul describes in Ephesians 4:11–12, if you are at home alone? How many apostles, prophets, evangelists, pastors and teachers are sleeping in, puttering in their garages or baking banana bread on Sunday morning instead of coming to the house of the Lord to help raise up more apostles, prophets, evangelists, pastors and teachers?

4. How else can you interpret Paul's instructions in 1 Corinthians 14 about how to use spiritual gifts in a church service except to mean that you are supposed to go to church and use your spiritual gifts in a service? (And I hope your church is like Eastgate and lets you!)

5. How do you "spur one another on toward love and good deeds" (Hebrews 10:24 NIV) sitting at home watching TV church?

6. How can you possibly read Deuteronomy 31:12 (ERV), "Assemble the people, the men and the women and the little ones, and thy stranger that is within thy gates, that they may hear, and that they may learn," and not envision

men, women, children and visitors assembling at a church service to learn?

7. How do you read Hebrews 10:25 (BSB), "Let us not neglect meeting together," and not believe in church "meetings"?

8. Why would Paul go to such great lengths in 1 Corinthians 12 to compare us to a body and warn us to stay connected as one if we were free to stay home and do our own thing?

9. How can pastors obey the mandate in 1 Peter 5:2 (ISV) to "be shepherds of God's flock that is among you, watching over it" if they do not know who or where their sheep are?

10. Why would Jesus say in Matthew 16:18 that He would build His Church (and that the gates of hell would not prevail against it) if He just wanted us to scatter in isolation and never convene?

The obvious answers to those questions are "You can't," "They can't" or "He didn't"! You can study the entire New Testament and not find a single lone-ranger Christian. The Christians of the Bible were interconnected and interdependent. And the epistles did not single out Christians about their own needs; rather they always referred to a church or community the recipient was connected to or where the letter would be read, and they included greetings to other believers there. You always read of the apostles mentioning churches at large, not investing their time in training free-spirited loners.

Christians are referred to as "sheep" and pastors as "shepherds" or "undershepherds" for good reason. Sheep are known to be senseless, smelly, stupid animals. That fence is their protection, not their restriction. They will follow something (or someone) right off a cliff unless stopped. Distracted sheep will never see a wolf until it is too late, and once they do they cannot outrun it. They need protection. Shepherds love to give it. It is safer in the sheepfold.

Yes, I know that "the most High dwelleth not in temples made with hands" (Acts 7:48 KJV; see also Acts 17:24), that your body is now the temple of God (1 Corinthians 3:9, 16, 17; 6:19–20; Ephesians 2:20–22) and that God says, "What house will ye build me?" (Acts 7:49 KJV). We *are* the Church. I get it. But gathering together in a building does not negate that. If you let Scripture interpret Scripture, it conveys as a whole that isolationism is contrary to God's will for His people. Besides, I do not *have to* go to church. I get to. "I was glad when they said to me, 'Let us go to the house of the LORD!'" (Psalm 122:1).

Distracted sheep will never see a wolf until it is too late, and once they do they cannot outrun it. They need protection. Shepherds love to give it. It is safer in the sheepfold.

If you still think regular church attendance is optional, then you are deceived. Jesus is returning for one matured Bride, not a bunch of little infantile ones. Church attendance is about winning the lost, yes, and about fellowship and service, yes, but mainly about readying yourself for the most spectacular wedding in history, of which you are a main participant.

Spiritually healthy people attend church at least weekly. Do you go 30 percent of the time, 60 percent or 100 percent? Do you want a 100 percent successful life? Then aim to attend church 100 percent of the time. Evidently, Nigeria tops the list of church attendance by nation, with weekly attendance at 89 percent, and Russia is at the bottom at 2 percent. How often does your household go? Once a month? Twice? Three times a month? Friend, I was in church three times *a week* growing up. My roots go so deeply in Christ and His Church that they can never be severed as long as I stay rooted. I am fielding blessings left and right today that I *know* are a direct result of my parents taking me to church when I was young. I do not remember a single, solitary Sunday when we were not at church as a family. I never knew it was an option to stay home, and I have heard

69

my mother say the same about her upbringing. It has been my life's work to replicate that priority in my own children and grandchildren by planting them firmly in the house of the Lord. "Those that be planted in the house of the LORD shall flourish in the courts of our God" (Psalm 92:13 KJV).

Healthy Habit Helpers

1. Do you attend church at least weekly? Why or why not? Do you see how Scripture champions this idea? What changes can you make beginning this week?

_____

_____

_____

_____

Now put your hand on your heart and pray this aloud with me:

God, thank You for the church where You have called me to serve (or to go find). Grace my life to make attendance a priority, find where I can best serve there and do so with excellence. I declare in Jesus' name that the enemy will not have my Sundays or any other day of the week when I am to be at my church's family table. Thank You for Your Church. Amen.

7

Stay Put

I grew up in a great denomination that believed "once saved, always saved." I took great comfort in the fact that nothing could snatch me from God's hand, and I still do. But now that I have had friends and longtime ministry partners *jump out* of God's hand and renounce their Christianity, I have had to rethink my position on this. I do not like angry verse-slinging on this topic when the two sides come together in a heated debate; so, since I recently felt both sides rising up in me for a perhaps not heated but lively debate, I decided to argue with myself and resolve this once and for all, with Scripture's assistance. (It also meant I was going to win one way or the other!)

Let me be clear: I do not believe we can "lose" our salvation. My question has never been about losing it but about giving it away. To my surprise, the verses I found corroborating the possibility of denying Christ and falling from faith after salvation outnumbered the verses indicating "once saved, always saved" by *ten times*. I found three Scriptures that *implied* it is not possible to return to an unsaved status after being saved, but I found thirty that state forthrightly it is. Here are the first dozen (emphasis mine):

71

Now the Spirit expressly says that in later times *some will depart from the faith* by devoting themselves to deceitful spirits and teachings of demons.

1 Timothy 4:1

If anyone does not abide in me he is *thrown away like a branch* and withers; and the branches are gathered, thrown into the fire, and burned.

John 15:6

For false christs and false prophets will arise and perform great signs and wonders, so as to lead astray, if possible, *even the elect.*

Matthew 24:24

For if we go on sinning deliberately after receiving the knowledge of the truth, there *no longer remains a sacrifice for sins*, but a fearful expectation of judgment, and a fury of fire that will consume the adversaries.

Hebrews 10:27

If we endure, we will also reign with him; *if we deny him, he also will deny us*; if we are faithless, he remains faithful—for he cannot deny himself.[1]

2 Timothy 2:12–13

For freedom Christ has set us free; stand firm therefore, and do not submit again to a yoke of slavery. . . . You are *severed from Christ*, you who would be justified by the law; you have fallen away from grace.

Galatians 5:1, 4

If indeed you continue in the faith, stable and steadfast, not shifting from the hope of the gospel that you heard, which has

---

1. So we see there is a difference between faithlessness and outright denial.

been proclaimed in all creation under heaven, and of which I, Paul, became a minister.

Colossians 1:23

Take care, brothers, lest there be in any of you an evil, unbelieving heart, *leading you to fall away from the living God.* But exhort one another every day, as long as it is called "today," that none of you may be hardened by the deceitfulness of sin. For we share in Christ, if indeed we hold our original confidence firm to the end.

Hebrews 3:12–14

But I have this against you, that you have *abandoned the love you had at first.* Remember therefore from where you have fallen; repent, and do the works you did at first. If not, I will come to you and remove your lampstand from its place, unless you repent.

Revelation 2.4

For if, after they have escaped the defilements of the world through the knowledge of our Lord and Savior Jesus Christ, they are again entangled in them and overcome, the last state has become worse for them than the first. For it *would have been better for them never to have known the way of righteousness than after knowing it to turn back* from the holy commandment delivered to them.

2 Peter 2:20–21

For it is *impossible to restore again to repentance* those who have once been enlightened, who have tasted the heavenly gift, and have shared in the Holy Spirit, and have tasted the goodness of the word of God and the powers of the age to come, *if they then fall away,* since they are crucifying once again the Son of God to their own harm and holding him up to contempt.

Hebrews 6:4–6

But the one who *endures to the end* will be saved.

Matthew 24:13

Mercy! Those twelve passages are unnerving! Fearsome, but impossible to dodge scripturally. For those of you who are still skeptical, let's restate these verses in plain black and white:

- In later times some will depart from the faith.
- Some will not abide in Him, and their future is fire.
- Even some of the elect will be deceived.
- Jesus' sacrifice no longer remains for those who keep deliberately sinning after knowing the truth.
- If we deny Christ, He will deny us.
- If we do not stand firm, we can be severed from Christ and fall away from grace.
- Jesus wants to present us blameless to God, but we must continue in the faith and not shift from the hope of the Gospel.
- It is possible to fall away from the living God and we only share in Christ if we hold our original confidence firm to the end.
- If we abandon our first love (Jesus), He will remove our lampstand.
- If we are saved from our sins and then become entangled in them again, it is worse than our original state of sin; it would be better for us to have never known the way of righteousness.
- It is impossible for those who fall away to be restored again to repentance, because they continue to crucify the Son of God.
- Only those who endure to the end will actually be saved.

If those twelve passages (and the recap) are not enough to convince you that it is possible to be deceived and fall away from the living God, here are eighteen more to study. Each reinforces the idea that salvation is a process of endurance and puts an indisputable priority on obedience and faithfulness in order to remain in Christ. Yes, your soul was saved in its entirety on a certain date, but you work out that salvation with fear and trembling. In other words, it was "worked in" all at once but it is "worked out" by a process. Here are the additional eighteen passages:

James 5:19–20—It is possible to wander from the truth and have it lead to death for your soul.

Philippians 2:12–13—Your salvation must be worked out with fear and trembling.

2 Corinthians 13:5—Examine and test yourself to make sure you are staying in the faith and that Jesus is still in you!

Romans 11:19–22—God cut off faithless Israel, and He will cut you off, too, if you do not stand fast in the faith.

Mark 13:13; Matthew 10:22—Only those who endure to the end will be saved.

Galatians 5:19–21—Certain people will not inherit God's Kingdom if they stay in the flesh and do not live by His Spirit.

Matthew 7:21—Not everyone who calls God "Lord" will get to heaven.

Romans 2:6–8—If we do not obey the truth, there will be wrath and fury.

Romans 8:12–13—If we live by the flesh, we will die.

1 John 3:6–9—Do not be deceived; whoever makes a practice of sinning is of the devil. No one born of God makes a practice of sinning.

Mark 16:16—If we do not believe, we come under condemnation.

John 3:36—If we do not obey, we will not see life.

1 John 5:16–17—All wrongdoing is sin, but there is sin that leads to death (implied *eternal* death).

1 John 5:18—If we are born of God, we do not keep sinning (deliberately). Only those born of God can be protected from the evil one.

Galatians 4:9—It is possible to turn back again to slavery.

Revelation 3:2–5—Only those who conquer will be clothed in white and are secure from not having their names blotted out of the Book of Life.

Now that I have given you thirty Scripture passages supporting the idea that it is possible to fall away from God and salvation, let me give you the three that I used growing up to support "once saved, always saved" (emphasis mine):

Who shall separate us from the love of Christ? Shall tribulation, or distress, or persecution, or famine, or nakedness, or danger, or sword? As it is written, "For your sake we are being killed all the day long; we are regarded as sheep to be slaughtered." No, in all these things we are more than conquerors through him who loved us. For I am sure that neither death nor life, nor angels nor rulers, nor things present nor things to come, nor powers, nor height nor depth, *nor anything else in all creation, will be able to separate us from the love of God* in Christ Jesus our Lord.

Romans 8:35–39

My sheep hear my voice, and I know them, and they follow me. I give them eternal life, and *they will never perish*, and no one will snatch them out of my hand. My Father, who has given them to me, is greater than all, and no one is able to snatch them out of the Father's hand. I and the Father are one.

John 10:27–30

For the gifts and the calling of God are irrevocable.

Romans 11:29

Suddenly, I am seeing the first one, Romans 8:35–39, through new eyes. Are you? It only says that nothing can separate us from God's *love*, which I believe fervently—but it mentions nothing about being separated from our salvation. There is a difference between love and salvation; if there were not, then God could have just loved us into heaven without needing to send Jesus to save us. So we can at least be comforted through this verse that even if we renounce our salvation, God will still love us. But that love does not override our God-given free will to renounce our salvation, and I have seen many do it.

As for the second passage, from John 10, Jesus makes sure we understand that once we follow Him, He will give us eternal life, we will never perish and no one will ever snatch us out of His hand. That is what happens when we follow Him—but what happens if we stop following Him? Here, He connects our protection from perishing with our willingness to follow Him. Furthermore, just because nothing can snatch us from His hand does *not* mean that we cannot jump out of His hand voluntarily. It is true that nobody could pull you from a vehicle speeding along at a hundred miles per hour, but that does not mean you are incapable of opening the door and jumping out yourself . . . to your death.

Let me be clear: Nobody can revoke or reverse your salvation. But it does appear that you yourself can abandon it. Proof of this comes later in John 15:6 (NIV 2011), when Jesus says, "If you do not remain in Me, you are like a branch that is thrown away and withers; such branches are picked up, thrown into the fire and burned." Friend, why on earth would Jesus warn us to remain in Him (or else be thrown into a fire) if we could not go anywhere else? That would be like chaining a person in a prison cell and asking him to remain there. You would waste your breath if he was unable to go anywhere. I believe this shows we do have a choice whether or not we remain in Christ.

Furthermore, just because nothing can snatch us from His hand does not mean that we cannot jump out of His hand voluntarily.

Finally, Romans 11:29 mentions that the gifts and calling of God are irrevocable. "Gift" in the Greek is *charisma*,[2] which means "favour, the gift of divine grace, the gift of faith, knowledge, holiness, virtue, the pardon of sin, extraordinary powers" and more. It does not mean "salvation," but it does include "the pardon of sin." The word translated "calling," which in the Greek is *klesis*,[3] means "a calling; invitation; divine invitation to embrace salvation." So we see that while "gifts and calling" do not mean "salvation," they do describe an invitation to the pardoning of sin.

So the invitation to the pardoning of sin is "irrevocable." What does that mean? "Irrevocable" is the Greek word *ametameletos*[4] and means "unregretted" and "without repentance." The NLT says, "can never be withdrawn," and other major translations end with "are without repentance." Put together, Romans 11:29 actually means that God does not and will not

2. "Lexicon: Strong's G5486—*charisma*," Blue Letter Bible, accessed April 20, 2017, https://www.blueletterbible.org/lang/lexicon/lexicon.cfm?Strongs=G5486&t=KJV.

3. "Lexicon: Strong's G2821—*klēsis*," Blue Letter Bible, accessed April 20, 2017, https://www.blueletterbible.org/lang/lexicon/lexicon.cfm?Strongs=G2821&t=KJV.

4. "Lexicon: Strong's G278—*ametamelētos*," Blue Letter Bible, accessed April 20, 2017, https://www.blueletterbible.org/lang/lexicon/lexicon.cfm?Strongs=G278&t=KJV.

ever regret or be sorry for extending the invitation to us for the pardoning of sin. Even if we say no, or even if we say yes and then change our minds, He still does not regret the invitation. This does not mean, however, that once we have accepted the invitation to live forever in heaven, we cannot return the invitation before we get there.

I think I once had a hard time believing salvation could be renounced because, frankly, I had not seen anyone officially do it. If people seemed to, I decided that they had never really been saved to begin with. That or they were saved and just backslidden but still eternally secure. But when you see a long-time pastor—one who did great deeds, saw countless salvations, performed dramatic miracles, fed the poor and loved his family and flock—pridefully turn from Christ, entirely renounce his salvation and enter into a life of perversion, you have to rethink your doctrine. Jesus said in Matthew 24 that in the last days the love of many would grow cold and that even the elect would be deceived. I believe we are in those days.

I would never want to make you feel uncomfortable or pressure you to give up your "once saved, always saved" doctrine. But I will charge you to do the following: *Stay put.* Remain. Do not let your love grow cold or your lampstand be taken from you. Guard your salvation as if your eternal life depends on it, because it does.

Healthy Habit Helpers

1. Are you remaining in Christ? Do you know of anyone who has renounced his or her salvation or appeared to? Use the

space below to write the names of those you know who need prayer to "stay put":

_____

_____

Now put your hand over your heart and pray this aloud with me:

Jesus, I can never thank You enough for giving Your life for me so that, by asking You to dwell in my heart, I can partake in Your holiness and stand before a holy God, both here and for eternity. Help me to stay rooted in You and to endure to the end, and use me to influence others to do the same. In Your name, Jesus, Amen.

8

Accept No Substitutes

What do you think of when you hear the word *substitute*? Maybe you use a salt substitute for your food. Maybe a sugar substitute. Maybe you are a substitute teacher, or know one. Perhaps at some point you have had to scramble to find a recipe substitute, like when you forgot eggs at the store and had a cake to make by suppertime!

This healthy living habit is intended to shine a light on any spiritual substitutions in your life—people, places or things that have the potential of taking a seat in your spirit (or mind or body) that should be occupied solely by the Holy Spirit. The thing about substitutions is that that they are often totally acceptable and wildly celebrated by the masses. There are whole websites created just for egg substitute innovations. If I were a chicken browsing the web, I would be very, very worried. You and I know that there are still billions of egg eaters out there, but if you are not one of them, abundant wisdom from the webernet is there to persuade you that a mixture of vegetable oil, water and baking powder is a healthy substitute for an egg. Your cake will taste the same, and your friends will be impressed; but your body will be saying, "Hey, where's my protein, selenium, folate, biotin, calcium, cephalin, lecithin, pantothenic acid, vitamin B12, vitamin A, iodine, vitamin E, phosphorous, iron, thiamine, zinc and vitamin D?!" Better to just borrow eggs from a neighbor or go the extra mile and return to the store, follow the original recipe and give your friends a healthy cake (gluten free, obviously!).

I am at a disadvantage because I do not know what the bookmarked substitution websites are in your life—i.e., the established sources and authorities that you visit regularly for advice. Friends and familiar mindsets have told you it is okay to have certain spiritual substitutions, or they may have convinced you that they are neither spiritual nor substitutions at all. Those voices in your ear are bound to be louder and more trusted than mine. So my job here is not to argue the morality or immorality of these substitutions but to awaken you to a zero-substitution policy in your life, whispering to you what perhaps no one else can, will or has been allowed to.

When I first prayed about writing this healthy living habit, I asked God for a title. Immediately, I heard in my spirit, *Accept No Substitutes*. I believe there is something important in the word *substitute* that God wants to say and warn us about. Let's look first at *Merriam-Webster's* definition: "To put or use (someone or something) in place of someone or something else; to do the job of someone else or serve the function of something else; to replace (one person or thing) with another."

So, if you are making a substitution of any kind, you are putting something to use in another's place, to do his or its job, effectively replacing him or it.

Let's dig a bit deeper into the word's origin (trust me, it is important): "'Substitute' has roots in fourteenth-century Middle English from the Anglo-French *substitut*, from Latin *substitutus*, with the past participle of *substituere*, which means, 'to put in place of.'"[1]

1. *Merriam-Webster's Collegiate Dictionary*, 11th ed., s.v. "substitute."

Breaking down the etymology further, *Merriam-Webster's* says *substitute* is a combination of *sub* and *statuere*:

sub: less than completely, perfectly, or normally

statuere: comes from the same root as the word *statute*, which means "a law, an act intended as a permanent rule"

That etymology is very important to our particular application, because, when coupled with the definition for *substitute*, and by merely replacing the word *someone* with any member of the Trinity, the definition of a "spiritual substitution" becomes this:

Something that is less than completely, perfectly or normally God's best for your life that is used in place of The Holy Spirit, does His job, serves a function He serves and replaces Jesus, intending to become a law and to set up permanent rule in your life.

How sobering! God has an opinion about that "thing" you turn to when in need of peace, comfort or companionship! It may not even be diabolical, just less than His complete, perfect best for you in that moment, and when you turn to it again and again and again, it eventually sets up permanent rule in your life.

So what are some of these substitutions? They can be anything. Literally anything. But over the last 25 years in ministry, I have noticed a definite top five. And only in the last 13 years as senior pastors have we had front-row seats in people's confidential lives and learned the patterns. These are in no order, and some require less explanation than others. And, again, this is not a forum to argue that these are moral or immoral, but that they are potentially dangerous spiritual substitutions when you are in need of peace, comfort or companionship.

1. **Food.** Sin first entered the world through appetite. Adam and Eve ate the forbidden fruit. Esau sold his birthright for a pot of stew. The Israelites grumbled when they got tired of the desert menu. Jesus passed the appetite test by refusing to turn stones into bread when tempted. Food is intimately linked to the spirit, as evidenced by what happens when we remove it and fast. Therefore, in times of discontent over anything, great or small, never let food do God's job, which is to comfort you. It can be the healthiest of food, created on day three in the Garden of Eden, but if you turn to it instead of to God in a moment of need, it can have deadly effects on your future. Even one meal. Ask Eve.

2. **Alcohol (and other substances).** Like food, alcohol is totally legal. But as pastors, we have seen it destroy the lives of countless nonalcoholics, not to mention alcoholics. We have seen uncharacteristically poor decisions made while under its influence (drunk or not): virginities lost, babies conceived, affairs had, marriages left, even death (including suicide). But there is no getting around the fact that Christians are sharply divided on their interpretations of what Scripture says about the topic, and sometimes even sharply divided within their own families. For example, I am a winemaker's daughter. I have stomped out my father's homegrown grapes for him, and yet I have never had a glass of wine. The short version of the story involves a rude awakening in 1985 that resulted in us ridding our home of alcohol and touching not a drop since; the longer version is in a free e-book that is available for download in my website's online store.[2] *Wine and Spirits* is a story of three biased characters, the Prohibitionist, the Moderationist and the Abstentionist, but the book itself is unbiased,

2. Laura Harris Smith, *Wine and Spirits*, 2016, http://www.LauraHarrisSmith.com/store.html.

with more research gathered from science, statistics and Scripture than any other publication I have ever seen on the issue. The reader takes in each chapter's information and then listens to the Prohibitionist, Moderationist and Abstentionist process it all. Many people mistake me for a prohibitionist, but I am not. I just want to see fewer people substituting the Holy Spirit's comfort with the fruit of the vine or field. Many other substances besides alcohol can be abused (including nicotine), some legal and some illegal, but all are potentially dangerous substitutions that can compromise one's spirit while opening the door to addiction and becoming a "permanent rule" in your life.

3. **Yoga or New Age Meditation.** Yoga is not just body-strengthening stretches or mind-calming exercises any more than expressive Christian worship is just vocal and arm exercises. Yoga—in its many varieties and schools—is an ancient spiritual discipline of the Hindu and Buddhist religions. According to meditation educator Yogi Padma,[3] yoga "exercises" cannot be separated from this spiritual component. When she came from India to America, she explains, she was

> amazed to see photos of North Americans practicing power yoga poses and talking about how yoga is good for getting a fit body. . . . In India, yoga has been studied and practiced for thousands of years, but it's not the look of the physical body that is the main aim of yoga there.

In truth, the poses themselves are offerings to the more than 330 million Hindu gods,[4] so for a Christian to remove

3. Padma (Marla Stewart), "What Is the Meaning of Yoga?," *Gaia*, October 2, 2012, https://www.gaia.com/article/what-meaning-yoga.
4. Laura Bagby, "Should Christians Do Yoga?," *CBN News*, accessed April 20, 2017, http://www1.cbn.com/700club/should-christians-do-yoga.

all Eastern New Age language from the discipline, replace it with biblical principles and call it "Christian yoga" is naïve, comparable to calling yourself a Christian Buddhist or a Christian Hindu. You may claim it with the purest of intentions, but the 330 million gods who lay legal claim to those poses you are doing are still honored and conjured every time you conform your body to them. You are being yoked to these spirits—in Sanskrit, in fact, the word *yoga* means "yoke" or "to yoke" (control, join, union). Surely the only way a Christian can fall for this type of practice is because in the early instruction of it, one of yoga's main concepts is introduced, which is to "empty the mind." The most famous yoga pose of all—the tree pose (vrikshasana[5])—is a remembrance of Queen Sita, who was kidnapped by the demon king Ravana, who threatened that he would cook and eat her if she continually refused him. She sat by a tree, breathed and sent her thoughts and love into the tree to become reunited with her true love. In the words of Kausthub Desikachar, grandson of revered Indian yoga master T. K. V. Krishnamacharya, "By meditating on these characters, we hope that we might come to embody some of their attributes."[6]

Embody? My body is off-limits to any other spirit but the Holy Spirit, and yours should be, too. I know this is hard for some of you to hear, but I implore you to resist offense right now. To say that you have nothing to do with the demons these poses salute simply because you do not mention them or think about them during yoga is

5. Zo Newell, Ph.D., "The Mythology behind Vrikshasana (Tree Pose)," *Yoga International*, January 26, 2015, https://yogainternational.com/article/view/the-mythology-behind-vrikshasana-tree-pose.

6. "Ancient Superheros," *Citta Vrtti Nirodhah: A Yoga Journal* (blog), August 16, 2013, https://cittavrttinirodhah.wordpress.com/2013/08/16/virabhadra-vasistha-vishvamitra-astavakra-goraksha-matsyendra/.

childlike and foolish. If in the early 1940s you had chosen as a curious young revolutionist to attend a Nazi rally and, being unsure of your allegiances, opted not to say, "Heil Hitler," when you gave the Nazi salute, what do you think Adolf Hitler and everyone around you would have thought of your physical participation? That salute would have been seen by Hitler and the spirits that controlled him as an offering of your devotion to him . . . and to them. Likewise, the demons themselves assume you are welcoming them when you strike any yoga pose. Your heart is entirely free of that motive, but remember: One of the concepts introduced early in yoga is to "empty the mind," and having done that, I believe, many Christians unknowingly invite deceiving spirits in. As a Christian, you are not to "empty your mind" but to be renewed by the transforming of it and to take every thought captive to the obedience of Christ. Emptying it leaves it vacant and vulnerable. Yoga—the act of being yoked—is just the beginning. That is the furthest thing from your mind when you are excitedly buying your yoga mat, selecting your yoga clothes and anticipating your new relaxed state, but once you yoke yourself to these spirits and this discipline, a door to deception opens in the spirit realm, and your life will take a turn, one poor decision at a time. Do not be unequally yoked (2 Corinthians 6:14). Consider Matthew 11:29–30 (NIV) instead: "Take my yoke upon you and learn from me, for I am gentle and humble in heart, and you will find rest for your souls. For my yoke is easy and my burden is light."

4. **Relationships.** Of all substitutions, this one is the easiest to mistake as an acceptable replacement for turning to God when in need of peace, comfort or companionship. Even the most godly spouse, parent, pastor, best friend

or children can eclipse God. There is nothing wrong with those relationships—and they are gifts from heaven—but the key is to "know thyself well" and not to turn to these gifts when you should turn to the Giver of them in your moments of greatest need.

5. **Busyness/Work/Ministry.** This one requires very little explanation. You know whether or not you are a workaholic. I am. Because I believe firmly in the rule of God first, family second and ministry third, however, I decided long ago to use that work ethic to my advantage and also to work very hard at rest, play and family togetherness. I do. As a result, my life is well-balanced and my work (which involves being here with you right now) is a light and easy burden to me and to those who love me and honor Christ.

I am certain there are other potential spiritual substitutions I have left out, but these five are the ones that we repeatedly battle as pastors. And somebody will argue that each of the five is undeserving of appearing on this list. My advice stands. Accept no substitutes.

I also find it interesting that from the word *statuere* comes the word *statue*. A statue sounds an awful lot like an idol, wouldn't you say? Put together, I believe this word *substitute* carries with it a strong warning against subtle imposters whose end goals are to set up permanent rule in your life and be erected as full-blown idols. Spiritually healthy people do not tolerate this in their lives.

"Thou shalt have no other gods before me" (Exodus 20:3 KJV).

Healthy Habit Helpers

1. In this "top five" list I have assembled from my years in ministry, are any of these spiritual substitutions potential

stumbling blocks to you? If not, name some that could be. We will ask the Holy Spirit to enlighten and deliver you.

_____

_____

_____

Now put your hand over your heart and pray this aloud with me:

Oh, great God, I ask Your forgiveness for any spiritual sub-stitutions I have allowed in my life. Forgive me for anything that took Your place, was allowed to do Your job, functioned in Your stead and set up permanent rule in my body, mind or spirit. Deliver me from these distractions. You alone are my Comforter, my Prince of Peace and my Great Companion. I renounce all counterfeits now, in Jesus' name, and vow to You that I will rid my life entirely of these substitutions. Grace me now, O God. In Your name, Amen.

9

Take Leaps of Faith

Spiritually healthy people understand risk. They are fearless—not irresponsible, but hopeful that the choices they make after much prayer and counsel will bear good fruit, so they learn to operate with less hesitation and worry. They take chances but are not reckless. They are grounded in God's Word and sensitive to His Holy Spirit, and they would never make a leap that contradicted Scripture and wise counsel (which they surround themselves with and are submitted to). But these people do not have to be pushed to step out on a limb and trust God. They seem to be instinctively brave and positive.

If you merely wake up every day, go to work, do your job to the best of your abilities, come home, engage in a hobby or time with loved ones, go to sleep and get up to do it all over again, you are never engaging your supernatural self. There is a sleeping faith giant inside of you that wants to waken and make decisions for you. That faith giant is none other than the Holy Spirit. He knows exactly what will make you happy and fulfilled. He knows exactly when you were conceived in your mother's womb and why. The Holy Spirit does not want you to live the same dull year 85 times and call it a life. Remember that He has to endure that dull life with you! Not that there is anything wrong with staying in the same profession for fifty years and retiring with a handsome pension—what I am describing far transcends the type of job you do and addresses how and why you do it. Are you doing your job with a temporal mindset or an eternal one? The temporally minded think of activities pertaining to the day to day of life. The eternally minded think about where others are spending their afterlives and filter daily activities through that grid.

One of my favorite verses on faith is Romans 10:17 (KJV): "So then faith cometh by hearing, and hearing by the word of God." The reason it is one of my favorites is twofold. First, it makes the connection between faith and Scripture crystal clear, which is key if you are going to have a well-balanced definition of faith. Faith without scriptural support is just being a daredevil. Without a biblical definition of faith you will start

> The Holy Spirit does not want you to live the same dull year 85 times and call it a life. Remember that He has to endure that dull life with you!

making decisions that embarrass both you and God. But with it you can move mountains, glorify Him and enjoy an adventurous life.

The second reason I love Romans 10:17 is that it shows the connection between faith and hearing. Hearing God's Word is where faith is born! It is where your doubt dissolves and hope arises. Hebrews 4:12 explains the reason for this, which is that the Word of God is alive! It is living and active! By just reading it with your eyes, you are empowering it to divide your soul from your spirit like a two-edged sword, so just imagine what *hearing* it read aloud accomplishes, especially if you are the one doing the speaking! So I have gathered a top ten list of faith passages for you (including Romans 10:17), and I want you to read them *aloud*. You need to hear yourself read them, and you need to hear them often.

"Now faith is the assurance of things hoped for, the conviction of things not seen" (Hebrews 11:1).

"And whatever you ask in prayer, you will receive, if you have faith" (Matthew 21:22).

"So faith comes from hearing, and hearing through the word of Christ" (Romans 10:17).

"And without faith it is impossible to please him, for whoever would draw near to God must believe that he exists and that he rewards those who seek him" (Hebrews 11:6).

"You believe that God is one; you do well. Even the demons believe—and shudder!" (James 2:19).

"For nothing will be impossible with God" (Luke 1:37).

"For we walk by faith, not by sight" (2 Corinthians 5:7).

"And Jesus said to him, 'If you can! All things are possible for one who believes.' Immediately the father of the child cried out and said, 'I believe; help my unbelief!'" (Mark 9:23–24).

"The apostles said to the Lord, 'Increase our faith!'" (Luke 17:5).

"Truly I say to you, if you have faith and do not doubt, you will not only do what was done to the fig tree, but even if you say to this mountain, 'Be taken up and cast into the sea,' it will happen. And all things you ask in prayer, believing, you will receive" (Matthew 21:21–22 NASB).

I challenge you to memorize these ten faith passages. They are short, making them easy to remember and recite daily. If you will do that, you will see a huge difference in your faith level. You will notice big changes in your decision making.

You will notice that the first verse on my list is Hebrews 11:1. In the New King James Version, it reads, "Now faith is the substance of things hoped for, the evidence of things not seen." This verse first came alive for me in my early twenties, when my husband and I were members of a wonderful Baptist church in Nashville pastored by Dr. William Roy Fisher and his wife, Yvonne. They were an amazing shepherd and shepherdess to their sheep, and I will never forget the first Sunday he preached on this verse. Whereas most sermons I had heard on Hebrews 11:1 focused on the key phrases of *the substance of things hoped for* and *the evidence of things not seen*, Dr. Fisher's focused on the first two words: *Now faith*. He challenged us to let our faith move us toward action ("Faith without works is dead") and never to wait or waver on trusting God. He even had lapel pins made for the whole congregation that read *NOWfaith*, with *NOW* in big red letters. It sparked a faith movement in our church. It sparked a faith movement in *me*! I still own that pin and wear it on days when I want to remind myself and others to choose faith, and so it is fitting that I am wearing it while writing this commentary.

Your faith has to be all or nothing. Doubt and faith cannot share the stage. In my opinion, you are either an atheist or a faitheist. You pick.

I wrote this poem almost twenty years ago, during a time when my faith was being tested during a difficult seven-year trial that I refer to as the "long obedience." This poem was written in year two, and I thought I could not go on another day. Had I known I had five years left, I might have set down my pen, lain down and died. I was learning the lessons of walking by faith and not by sight (2 Corinthians 5:7). The poem is the voice of a person confronting her doubts and realizing that one day she would go on to share with others the blind faith she was owning right at that moment. And she did.

Faith

Feeling my way along the walls
hoping that this will be
the very last corner I have to crawl
pretending that I can see

How did I get here on the ground
when before I was standing firm
Somehow I fell down, and now I resound
of another humbling term

It's dark in this place where no eye can see
where hope is the sole ray that beams
But some say that hope in faith's recipe
wakes the substance of all things yet seen

This room is much larger than at my first glance
when I first launched the search for the light
And I will say my senses have all been enhanced
as I've walked all this way without sight

Still I know the day nears when the lights will come on
Heaven's wiring has destined my hand
to map out this room 'til the walls are all gone
and enlighten those left where I stand

It's dark in this place where no eye can see
where hope is the sole ray that beams
But some say that hope in faith's recipe
wakes the substance of all things yet seen

© *Laura Harris Smith*

Healthy Habit Helpers

1. Name three areas in which you need to ask God to boost your faith:

_____

_____

_____

_____

Now put your hand over your heart and pray this aloud
with me:

*God, even as I am speaking this prayer out loud, You see into
my heart. You know why I make the decisions I do and the
fears that prevent me from making more faith-filled ones. I
reject all doubt and ask for Your grace to live a doubt-free
life. I receive a supernatural deposit of Your faith for these
three areas of my life right now, and I expect great things
are coming in them. In Your name, Jesus, Amen.*

10

Have a Come-to-Jesus Meeting

You know, neither the supernatural, nor prayer, nor the Spirit, scriptures, church or faith is going to mean anything to you if you have not experienced the transformation of salvation. Have you? You can know for sure. Ask yourself these three questions:

1. Did you pray for it?
2. Did you change after it?
3. Do you tell anyone about it?

I know these may seem like overly simplistic and irrelevantly shallow questions, but they cut to the heart of the matter. Let's dissect each one:

Did You Pray for It?

On what date did you pray and give your life to Jesus Christ? You should know. Just like you can point to an exact date for your birthday or anniversary, it is important that you remember the date when you made this life-changing decision. If you were too young to mark it on a calendar, perhaps you can ask a family member or at least recall a certain season and year. It is important to reflect on that decision at the same time each year, taking a personal inventory and marking what God has done for you. For me, that date was June 22, 1975. The bottom line is, make sure you understood a few crucial themes and meant them when you prayed them. What are those salvation themes?

In my early years, I learned quickly in church about what we called the "Romans road." It was a series of simple verses extracted from a long letter that Paul wrote about three decades after Jesus' resurrection to the Italians, Greeks, Jews and other Roman citizens who were dispersed among about five house churches in Rome. Just a little history here to make you appreciate the letter more fully: Romans was not one of Paul's prison epistles, and it was his longest, so he had to invest personally to hire a scribe (Romans 16:22, "I Tertius, who wrote this letter, greet you in the Lord.") for a job that is estimated to have taken eleven hours of dictation. The average papyrus letter was 87 words. Paul's average letter was 2,495 words. But this letter to the Romans is 7,114 words! So add to the scribe's labor the enormous amount of papyrus that was required for the mammoth job, and scholars have estimated the total cost of this letter to be 20.68 denarii, or $2,275 U.S. dollars.[1] In this light, we can safely say that the book of Romans was not a casual undertaking but a calculated, sophisticated defense of something. But what?

On what date did you pray and give your life to Jesus Christ? You should know.

1. Craig Keener, Ph.D., "Paul's Crafting of the Book of Romans—the $2275 Letter!," *Bible Background Research and Commentary*, December 19, 2011, http://www.craigkeener.com/pauls-crafting-of-the-book-of-romans-the-2275-letter/.

Clearly, Romans is a detailed, straightforward explanation of how salvation comes only through Jesus Christ. You might argue that $2,275 is worth investing into the billions of believers who have benefited from its words, but Paul had no reason to imagine such Kingdom success! He probably just thought he was writing a simple yet important letter to a minister who would share it with five house churches. What a word genius Paul was. How inspired by the Holy Spirit he was! There must be power in those words. Divine power. So it should make us appreciate the Romans road salvation themes even more. Here are the Cliffs Notes:

- **Everyone needs salvation: Romans 3:23.** "For all have sinned, and come short of the glory of God" (KJV). This shows that none are innocent. (And Romans 3:10–18 gives a detailed picture of what our sin looks like.)
- **Jesus died for our salvation: Romans 5:8.** "But God demonstrates His own love toward us, in that while we were yet sinners, Christ died for us" (NASB).
- **Salvation is a gift from God: Romans 6:23.** "For the wages of sin is death; but the gift of God is eternal life through Jesus Christ our Lord" (KJV).
- **God saves all who call upon Him: Romans 10:9–10.** "If you confess with your mouth Jesus as Lord, and believe in your heart that God raised Him from the dead, you will be saved; for with the heart a person believes, resulting in righteousness, and with the mouth he confesses, resulting in salvation" (NASB). We must only believe with the heart and confess with the mouth. So simple! I believe this double mentioning of the "mouth" shows the importance of praying for salvation out loud. Romans 10:13 reinforces this: "For everyone who calls on the name of the Lord will be saved" (HCSB).

Some other versions of the Romans road include Romans 4:5 (righteousness comes through faith), Romans 5:1 (we now have peace with God) and Romans 11:6 (we are saved by grace).

Wow. All of this—the thorough, unabridged message and the sacrifice it took to deliver it—makes me want to devour the whole book of Romans right now! I hope you will appreciate the gold nuggets within it, among which is the Romans road plan of salvation. And, more importantly, make sure that you have confessed these verses and truths with your mouth, marking the date when you do.

Did You Change after It?

Whereas question #1 could be answered by only you, this one might best be answered by those around you. Would those who knew you before you were saved say you were different afterward? I was a different ten-year-old after my decision for Christ. Beforehand, I had become "sad" and started to see a child psychologist; afterward I was filled with joy and did not need the antidepressants prescribed for me. What is your transformation story? Would those who know you today say you are still changed, or have you reverted to old behaviors from which Christ rescued you? When you come to Jesus, He does not clean up your life. He gives you a new one; thus, you are a new creation, which is why salvation is often referred to as being "born again." The Bible refers to it as the "new nature." Listen to these Scriptures, which convince us about the new creation (emphases mine):

> Therefore, if anyone is in Christ, *he is a new creation*. The old has passed away; behold, the new has come.
>
> 2 Corinthians 5:17

99

Seeing that you *have put off the old self* with its practices and have *put on the new self*, which is being renewed in knowledge after the image of its Creator.

Colossians 3:9–10

To *put off your old self*, which belongs to your former manner of life and is corrupt through deceitful desires, and to *be renewed* in the spirit of your minds, and to *put on the new self*, created after the likeness of God in true righteousness and holiness.

Ephesians 4:22–24

I have been crucified with Christ. *It is no longer I who live, but Christ* who lives in me. And the life I now live in the flesh I live by faith in the Son of God, who loved me and gave himself for me.

Galatians 2:20

We were buried therefore with him by baptism into death, in order that, just as Christ was raised from the dead by the glory of the Father, we too might *walk in newness of life.*

Romans 6:4

For neither circumcision counts for anything, nor uncircumcision, *but a new creation.*

Galatians 6:15

If nothing at all about you changed after you prayed and asked God to give you new life, then either you did not take the prayer seriously, you did not nourish your faith afterward and fell away or you need deliverance prayer to go to a new level in your sanctification process. Salvation does not come through works, but we do work out our salvation with fear and trembling (Philippians 2:12). Consider asking your church leaders for deliverance prayer: meeting with you in a private setting to discuss your past, breaking off whatever is holding you back from being the new person God has created you to be. He paid a great price for your new life and wants you to live it to the fullest!

Do You Tell Anyone about It?

This is the simplest question of all. If you have truly changed and become a new creature, not only does everyone notice it, but you cannot quit talking about it! Think back to how you first felt when you came to Jesus, or how you felt when you were closest to Him. Surely you told people about it. If you no longer do (or do not as much), you must ask yourself why. Be honest. If you had the cure for cancer, would you not feel compelled and excited to share it with every cancer patient you knew? Well, you do have the cure for not only cancer, but for whatever ails mankind—body, mind or spirit. If you truly believe in the Gospel message, you will want to give it away. You will live, sleep, eat and breathe evangelism. Listen to these verses that command us to share our faith (emphases mine):

> *Always be prepared to give an answer* to everyone who asks you to give the reason for the hope that you have.
>
> 1 Peter 3:15 NIV

> He said to them, "*Go into all the world and preach the good news* to all creation. Whoever believes and is baptized will be saved, but whoever does not believe will be condemned."
>
> Mark 16:15–16 NIV

> And I pray that the *sharing of your faith may become effective* for the full knowledge of every good thing that is in us for the sake of Christ.
>
> Philemon 6

Each day proclaim the good news that he saves. Publish his glorious deeds among the nations. Tell everyone about the amazing things he does.

Psalm 96:2–3 NLT

I am not ashamed of the gospel, because it is the power of God for the salvation of everyone who believes.

Romans 1:16 NIV

I tell you, whoever acknowledges me before men, the Son of Man will also acknowledge him before the angels of God. But he who disowns me before men will be disowned before the angels of God.

Luke 12:8–9 NIV

Woe to me if I do not preach the gospel!

1 Corinthians 9:16

I hope you see that you can know for sure if you have genuinely had a come-to-Jesus moment in your life. If you have any doubts at all, that ends today. I invite you to contemplate the following questions and pray with me afterward.

Healthy Habit Helpers

1. Do you know for sure that you have prayed to receive salvation? (Not a decision by your parents or your church, but by you, yourself.) On what date did you do so, and what changes did you notice in yourself?

_____

_____

_____

2. Do you speak often to others about your faith in Jesus Christ (not just God)? If not, why?

_____

_____

_____

Now put your hand on your heart and pray this aloud with me:

Jesus, I can never thank You enough for giving Your life for me, so that by asking You to dwell in my heart I can partake in Your holiness and stand before a holy God, both here and for eternity. I can also never ask You enough to take control of my life and circumstances. I give You my all, today. Come into my life. Let it be evident to all that You are changing me and changing the world through me. Father, give me a new vocabulary that I might share my faith with people in a relevant way without fear, and give people ears to hear the message You are giving me to speak to them. I ask all of this in Your name, Jesus, Amen.

Section 2

The Top 10 Healthy Living Habits for Your *Mind*

1

Get It Together

Organization is a scary word for some. Are you one of them? Do you freak out when the doorbell rings because of the condition of your home? Do you regularly hide certain areas from even extended family who visit? Do you have specific cabinets you pray no one will open, or that you yourself dread accessing? We all have places we "tuck" things from time to time, but if your whole house is "tucked" and you often cannot find things, or your idea of cleaning is to organize your clutter, something is wrong. Emotionally healthy people are organized, because a cluttered house is a symptom of a cluttered mind.

I love organization mainly because I hate wasting time, and there is no bigger time waster than disorganization. When you cannot find a piece of clothing, you are late for an appointment. When you trip over your piles, you get injured. When you cannot find a file on your computer, you miss a deadline.

107

Every room in your home consists of two things: a space and a schedule. You are in your kitchen around the same time each day. Home office, same thing. You spend one-third of your life in your bedroom, etc. We will start in these rooms in this commentary, since they are crucial. You need them organized so that the work you do in them can also be. In the next healthy living habit, "Plan Your Work and Work Your Plan," we will explore ways you can better organize the time you spend in those spaces and the activities that flow there.

Let's take a look at the top three spaces people find difficult to organize. Each space, when organized, can actually optimize your day and add hours to your week. I want to begin with kitchens and give you three easy tips that are going to put an end to mealtime madness.

Kitchens

- **Alphabetize your spice cabinet.** You will thank yourself every time you reach for a spice if you will just take ten minutes right now to alphabetize your spice cabinet. Guests will thank you, too (and be very impressed). If you do not have room for every letter of the alphabet on the front row, just create back rows, something you will have to do anyway with the Cs, due to the many spices that letter represents. While you are in there, the nutritionist in me advises you to throw out anything that is more than two years old because it has lost its nutritional value, not to mention its potency, thus disqualifying it as a "spice." From your *a*llspice to your *y*ellow mustard seeds (sorry, I file white pepper under *p*), an organized spice cabinet is a cook's best friend.

- **Purge all old plates, cups and flatware.** You have been reaching in that cup cabinet for so long that you do not even notice all the mismatched cups and glasses. But your guests do. And your family deserves better. Do yourself a favor and count how many you have of each type of glass or cup. If you have fewer than four of something, you need to part with it.

- **Organize your pantry and refrigerator.** Let each shelf have a segregated calling. One for cartons and jugs, one for fruits that need chilling, one for leftovers, etc. Same thing for your pantry. And aim for the majority of your meals to be prepared from the living foods in your refrigerator and not the "dead" foods in your pantry. This is tricky, because at the grocery store, the huge middle section of your store supplies your pantry with its dead food, whereas the foods along the perimeter of the store, where the electrical outlets are, go in your refrigerator. Let this motivate you. As you walk through the vast aisles of dead foods at your grocer, think of the size of your much smaller pantry and choose wisely and nutritionally.

Bedrooms

For all rooms in your house—especially bedrooms and closets—you have four options for parting with items as you clean and organize. If an item has gone unused for more than two years (most organizers say one year, so I am being generous), you can either sell it, gift it, trash it or donate it. As you are organizing each room, separating items into those four piles will make for speedy sorting. Some items, such as old family photos and baby books, are exempt, but be careful! If you are not disciplined, you will hang on to absolute junk in the name of sentiment. Since I am the most sentimental person I know (my husband says, "heavy on the 'mental'"), I will offer some friendly advice in the next healthy living habit, along with a funny story. For now, here are my tips for organization in your bedrooms.

- **Make your bedroom a sanctuary.** The original meaning of *sanctuary* is "a place of refuge or safety." When I was a TV host on the Shop At Home Network, my favorite segments were the bedding shows. The production assistants would decorate the set with a gorgeous bedroom suite with bedding to match, even curtains. And not only was the décor for sale but also the mattress and pillows underneath. I would say, "You spend a third of your life in bed; make your bedroom a sanctuary and enjoy it!" I say the same to you now.

- **Declutter.** A decluttered space lowers your stress. No piles in the corners. No ironing boards lying around. Only things in your dressers and chests that you need to access regularly. Only things *on* them that are aesthetically pleasing or full of good memories. And while you are making things more orderly, make your bed daily. It starts the day with a sense of accomplishment, feels more peaceful and inviting when you turn in at night and is better for your health! Why? You know all that dust that settles on your nightstand? It also settles on your bed each day, which you never dust; but making your bed at least keeps dust off your sheets and, therefore, off of you.

- **Put your bed on risers.** Needing extra storage space? Buy a set of risers and a bedskirt. Be very selective with what you put under your bed, but take advantage of that hidden real estate. I was able to store my collapsible treadmill, my massage table and all my nice framed pictures that need protection before I put them again on display.

Closets

In my busy, crowded household, my walk-in closet has always been the catchall for *anything* that *anybody* could not find a place for *anywhere else*. If it was too small for the garage or too sensitive to the elements, my closet became its home. Our closet is lined with shelves and has always been full of all manner of miscellany, from sheets to blankets to shoes to old treasures. But we went through a period when we needed an office for my husband but did not have an extra bedroom. So I cleared space in the closet, put in a small desk and a phone line and *voilà*! The "cloffice" was born. This only lasted a few years until a child moved out and a bedroom could be converted, but it taught me something very important: You *can* make room if you have to. Once the cloffice years were over and the desk removed, I set out to make every inch of that space count. Below are my tips for your closets, based on what I did to my own (throughout my whole house).

- **Add extra shelving.** We already had shelves above the closet racks where our clothes hung, but we added another shelf on top of those. We did this throughout the entire house and storage doubled!
- **Add drawers.** If possible, purchase plastic drawer units for your closets. In them you can store undergarments, scarves, T-shirts, socks and more.
- **Organize your clothes by color.** Whereas some people prefer their clothes organized in no system (or by season, at best), you can save huge amounts of time when getting dressed each day if you organize by color. I do the same with my shoes (on the shelves) and with my jewelry (in drawers with divider trays).

There are many things in life you cannot necessarily control—your salary, your health, your relationships—but you can *always* control your spaces. You can organize them in such a way that the work you do in them becomes more fluid and productive. We will discuss that in our next healthy living habit.

Healthy Habit Helpers

1. Name your major areas of disorganization and what you can do about them:

_____

_____

_____

Now put your hand on your heart and pray this aloud with me:

God, I have got to have change. I need order in my spaces and in my life. Give me the focus and discipline and creativity to get to work and get organized. In Jesus' name I pray, Amen.

2

Plan Your Work and Work Your Plan

In the previous healthy living habit, we discussed how emotionally healthy people organize their spaces. Now we will learn some tips for organizing the schedule in those spaces, meaning how to maximize your time in your newly organized areas. But first, some perils of not doing so.

A kitchen consists of cabinets, drawers, counter space and perhaps a pantry (or shelves). You have a limited amount of space to hold everything you will need for the preparation, serving, eating and cleanup of the more than one thousand meals you will eat in your home each year (that counts eating out one to two times each week). Every time you reach for an item to help you with one of those four purposes, you have the opportunity to save time or waste it. Let's say it takes you 45 minutes to prepare a meal, and during that time you touch one large appliance (range), two small appliances (convection toaster oven and mixer), six utensils and accessories (measuring spoons, measuring cup, paring knife, apple corer, whisk and colander), four spices and, of course, whatever foods you have purchased for that meal. But what if you cannot find the beaters for the mixer? It might take four minutes to find both of them in your disorganized utensils drawer, since they were not in the messy cabinet with the mixer. Then you waste another two minutes trying to find the right measuring spoon and another three digging through your spice cabinet looking for turmeric and cumin. Then it takes you three extra minutes to fish out those vegetables you bought that got shoved to the back of the fridge and never made it to the crisper, which, by the way, are now no longer fresh, leaving you to scramble to find a canned substitute for your recipe. Trouble is, you have no idea where your electric can opener is in that messy cabinet, and you really do not want to dig through the chaotic utensils drawer again for the manual one. So you recalibrate and start preparing a totally different dish, which costs another eight minutes. I am hoping by now you did not burn whatever else was cooking while you gave your full attention to all this searching, or even more time will be wasted. As it stands, you have lost twenty minutes due to disorganization.

That might not seem like a lot, but when multiplied by a thousand annual meals, that loss totals 20,000 minutes, or 333.3 hours. That is almost 14 days of your life in 1 year! Multiply that by 80 years and you lose 1,111 days, or *3 years* of your life! Think that is extreme? For some of you reading, it is, but for others (and you know who you are) it is not, because if it is not happening in the kitchen, it is happening in some other disorganized space in the house. Even if such time-devouring searching only happens to you a few times a week, you still lose more than 50 hours a year. Those are days chopped off of your life due to disorganization—days that could be spent

I guarantee that at the end of your life you will wish you had back all the hours, days, months and years you lost to disorganization.

relaxing by the fire, vacationing with your loved ones, praying and learning to hear God's voice better or *anything else besides needless searching.* I guarantee that at the end of your life you will wish you had back all the hours, days, months and years you lost to disorganization.

Let's start with some ideas on how you can save time in your newly organized spaces:

Kitchens

- **Use paper plates and cups.** Once I realized how much water my dishwasher was using to clean 24 plates of food a day (8 house residents × 3 meals a day), I felt much less guilty about regularly using paper plates and cups. I cannot replace river water, but I can plant a new tree every now and again to replenish the ones that make my paper plates. It also saves on cleanup time, which is a bonus!
- **"AMC!"** This is short for "after-meal chores." At Campsmith (our home), everyone had a postmeal responsibility. One would gather the trash, one would put away the leftovers, one would put away pantry items, one would gather silverware, one would wipe off the table and another would sweep. So after each meal, as everyone began to scatter, I would say, "AMC!" and everyone sprang into action. It took all of two minutes to clean up a meal for a family of eight.
- **Communal dinners and fellowship meals.** Some call them potlucks, Jacob's supper or covered-dish suppers. Call it what you may, they save endless time in the kitchen. When people wonder why I have been so willing to open up my home and entertain, I tell them it is because I learned the art of fellowship meals. In the early years of our church, when we did not yet have our own building and Eastgate

was very small (we started with only eighteen adults), we would host the fellowship meal at our house every Wednesday night. Everyone brought a dish and the church would provide drinks and disposable plates and utensils. Eventually we grew to the point that I had fifty people in my house each week, so we decided to form two groups, and our small-group ministry was born (now called "Connect Groups"). It has been fulfilling over the years to add more and more groups, knowing that it all started in my kitchen with a beautiful communal tradition.

Bedrooms and Offices

There is really no way for me to teach you to save time in your newly organized bedroom, because that would mean scrimping on sleep, which I do not want you to do! So, instead, I am going to show you simple tips for your home office (which may be in your bedroom), and you can also take these tips to your office away from home.

- **Find organized drawer space.** Believe it or not, I do not have a desk. I once had quite a large one in my bedroom but found that it kept me in the bedroom during the day, when I really needed to be with my children in the dining room homeschooling them. I have written twenty books—some published and some not—but only one of them was written entirely at a desk. My first book was written with a pen on twelve yellow legal pads! But not at a desk. I have been using laptops exclusively for the last twelve years or so, and therefore my lap is my desk, usually on a sofa. When I was on total bed rest writing *Seeing the Voice of God*, my bed was my desk. But while sofas and beds are wonderful places to recline and create, neither comes with

116

drawer space for organization. So, though I once had a long desk in my bedroom, now it is a regular long dresser, each drawer strategically filled with work-related items. Office supplies in one, laptop and accessories in another, etc. This has also forced me to run an entirely paperless ministry and business, which is great for the environment. My youngest is now a senior in high school and does not need me watching over her schooling, but I still want to be out there, and so I did not return to a desk in my room. I went with the dresser, which is part of our bedroom suite and looks more "bedroomish." If you were to walk in our home and look around, you would not even know that an author lives and works here. But she does! And quite productively, thanks to proper organization.

- **Organize your desktop!** Remember that even if you do not have a desk, if you have a computer, you have a desktop to keep tidy! Nobody likes to have someone look over her shoulder at her messy desktop. It gives the impression of disorder, and rightfully so. Take time every few days to clear and clean your desktop, just like you would the top of your desk in any office. And while you are at it, keep your email inbox clutter-free by unsubscribing from all spam and unsolicited mail that you wish would quit eating your time. Just take a few minutes every now and again to scroll to the bottom of unwanted emails and click "unsubscribe." You get added to mailing lists when you sign up or sign in to certain online companies, who then sell your email address for money. Occasional purging is required to rid your inbox of chaos.

- **Organize your day.** If you work away from home, then your blocks of time are set for you. If you work from home, you need to plan your work each day so that the day does not escape you and end with nothing to show for it. Either way, order your evenings and "downtime" to make sure you get plenty of R & R. And order your sleep schedule, too, so that you get regular deep, restorative sleep each night.

I once heard a funny anthem: "Procrastinators unite! Tomorrow!" Never wait to get organized, because, as we established, it wastes days and even years of your life. I was not always so organized, but having to run a large household that seemed to grow smaller as each child came forced me to learn.

In the previous healthy living habit, I promised to end with a humorous story about my difficulty parting with certain items. Remember: sell, donate, gift or trash it. But in some cases you will also be able to repurpose it, especially an item that holds great sentiment. And that leads to my story.

Never wait to get organized, because it wastes days and even years of your life.

When we remodeled our home years ago, we swapped out all the gold doorknobs for new brushed silver ones. But while removing each one, I kept envisioning the near twenty years' worth of memories they contained. How many tens of thousands of times had that pantry doorknob been turned by tiny (hungry) hands that grew into bigger hands? The occasional cleanings throughout the years had not dulled their collective memory. Suddenly, I could not part with it. I felt the same about the knobs from the three bedroom doors that our six children shared. So I wrapped them and stuck them in my closet—of course—only to be made fun of by said children (save one) whenever the topic arose. Finally, I realized that if those doorknobs were meant to make me happily nostalgic, they had to be *seen*. So I took them to my husband (a *very* creative carpenter) and asked him to mount them on wood for me. They now hang in my bedroom, where they display my many necklaces and keep them tangle-free. People see necklaces; I see knobs. And, occasionally, I imagine a tiny hand turning one of them, and it opens a door to my heart.

Healthy Habit Helpers

1. Name the rooms or activities you are going to better organize and the order in which you are going to organize them:

   _____

   _____

   _____

Now put your hand on your heart and pray this aloud with me:

Dear God, I feel the conviction to get it together and to plan my work. Inspire my mind and motivate my body to get going! Right now, I receive Your order to my home, work spaces and schedule. In Jesus' name, Amen!

3

Have a Heart
(and Mind Your Manners)

Whatever happened to being polite,
well mannered and pleasant and kind?
And why do we disregard life's dearest gestures
and hurriedly leave them behind?

We used to say "Yes ma'am" and "No sir" and "Thank you"
and ask God to bless every sneeze
But now we're more bridled; we feel more entitled
and barely can muster a please

Stop your critiquing; please look at who's speaking
and lay down your phone for a while
Don't interrupt or be rudely abrupt;
watch your tone and for heaven's sake smile!

Don't be so driven, shake a hand if it's given
and please use said hand if you yawn
Take your neighbor a meal, ask his wife how she feels
and then when they're gone mow their lawn

And when on the road, save the rage, don't explode;
when parking be kind, have a heart
Let someone cut line, change a tire, pay a fine
and take back that stray shopping cart

Hold a door, feed the poor, take your friend to the store;
go above and beyond for your brother
And when on the bus and a baby does fuss
give your seat to that tired nursing mother

Remember my friend, don't ever drop in;
call first, then go ready to serve
Serve at church, while you're at it; don't be too dogmatic
and stay off your pastor's last nerve

Say "You're welcome" when thanked, and sorry when
*   spanked*
and know when to keep your lip zipped
Be on time when you dine, grab the tab as you gab
and don't jilt your waitress her tip

If we'd keep in mind to be gracious and kind
and when not, to make speedy amends
We'd never again bring grief to our kin
or find ourselves lacking in friends

© Laura Harris Smith

You know, if you would adopt just half the tips in this poem, you would be the most well-liked person around! And if we all did all of them, the world would be a less cranky place.

If you have not figured this out about me yet, I like lists. So I have one for you here, the top twenty common courtesies for emotionally healthy people, and these go a bit deeper than just saying thank you or please. These are blunt and in no particular order.

1. **Cool it on Facebook and Twitter.** There is a difference between having an opinion and being opinionated. We all

121

have that one person on our friend list whose posts give us an ulcerative feeling in our stomachs. Do not be that friend. I refrain from inflammatory posts to begin with, but I also have a little image that I drop into a conversation thread if people are arguing on my timeline that says, "Don't you type at me in that tone of voice." I have another meme of a goofy monkey (actually, a lemur) that reads, "Calm down, bro." (Google it! Use it!) Be courteous on all your socials, and your friends will love you for it.

2. **Acknowledge when spoken to.** When you are spoken to, whether the answer is yes, no or wait, *say it*. Clearly. Do not assume the speaker can read your mind or see you taking action (especially on the phone). You appear rude when you mumble or do not answer.

3. **When giving criticism, start with something positive.** You work hard on a meal, blog post, gift or project, and upon finishing you ask for feedback. Here comes the guy (or gal) who whips out his list of shortcomings. Do not be that person, either! Start with something nice or do not start at all.

4. **Tip well or stay home.** I cannot tell you how many times I have heard of Christians shortchanging their waiters or waitresses a tip and instead leaving some religious pamphlet. You might as well have stolen the food. Quit making God look bad. Bowing your head to pray before your meal and then leaving at least a 20 percent tip goes a long way with servers who need to see who Jesus is, and when mixed with encouraging conversation, even further.

5. **Ask people questions.** Nobody likes a conversation hog. Oh, I talk a lot, but I love to inquire about people's lives and learn what makes them tick (taking mental notes). My husband's mother, Jackie, is the conversation question queen. I have heard her step into the worlds of every one

of my children: "Now, tell me . . . how did you feel when you were doing that dance?" Or, "Okay, so, why did you choose those colors for your painting?" She is genuinely interested, and it shows. Her last name is even Curtis, which means "courteous." Fitting!

6. **Quit talking over people**—especially if they are older than you. Yield. Listen. Wait your turn. This is experience talking!

7. **Greet the day.** Years ago, when my kiddos were small, I remember making a conscious effort to greet them in the morning with "Good morning," or at least a "Morning"! As they grew, they began to initiate it and still do today. Each day is special. Start it special with your own traditions. If you live alone, take this healthy living habit to work.

8. **Reward the little guy.** Probably the most frequent visitor to your house is your postman. Or garbage guy. When is the last time you showed them a kind gesture? My daughter, Jeorgi, bakes cookies for our postman. My husband sometimes takes bottles of cool water out to our garbage collectors. Years ago, when we got in a financial pinch with a growing household and added extra bins for collection (but had not paid), they just emptied them weekly for us anyway and never billed us a dime. Giving pays off!

9. **Say you're sorry.** Go first. God can always give you something to say you are sorry for to begin the dialogue. If it is not reciprocated, no worries. The blessing will come to you directly from God because you humbled yourself.

10. **Dress discreetly at church.** Yes, everywhere else, too. But you have no idea how many women's shirts I have gently "yanked" up to cover cleavage or yanked down to cover their backsides at an altar. Sometimes wardrobe malfunctions happen and cannot be helped, and I understand that,

but both men and women should think of others when preparing themselves for church, beginning with modest clothing.

11. **Receive a compliment.** The next time someone says something kind about you, resist the urge to roll your eyes and defer the attention. Say thank you. Just smile if that is all you can manage, but stop arguing with your encouragers! And, ladies, it is most likely not sexual harassment if a gentleman discreetly compliments you. Discern intentions, but try not to punish the good guys.

12. **Lend a helping hand.** I mention a lot of ideas in the poem that opens this healthy living habit, but here is a cool story: I was once in line at a famous author's book signing and had been there for more than an hour, with at least that to go. A couple in line behind us opened up to us that it was their anniversary and that they had driven five hours to get there, had called ahead and been told not to bother getting there early—and that they had paid two hundred dollars each for tickets to a concert that had now started without them. While my husband chatted with them, I dismissed myself, made my way to the front of the line and pled their case to the author's assistant. Without hesitation she told me to bring them to her, and I did. You should have seen their faces when I told them they could skip the line! The lady was crying and they thanked and hugged me. I honestly enjoyed that more than meeting the author—even though that was magnificently unforgettable, too. It is definitely better to give than receive!

13. **Encourage publicly.** Know someone who really needs encouraging? Ding your glass with your fork at a restaurant and tell the world how great he is. Announce good news for her in class, at church or on the bus. Tag him in a social media post with a picture that shows the world his

winning smile. Have a heart and show the world someone else's.

14. **Come clean.** Or, I should say, "*Go* clean." Before leaving the house, make sure you shower, brush your teeth, apply deodorant, have on freshly washed clothes and have given attention to other personal grooming, such as shaving, makeup and hair (whichever applies to you). A good friend will tell you if your refusal to do these things is ruining your reputation and their concentration, but in case you do not have a good friend (or a brave one), here I am.

15. **Be a gentleman (guys).** Open her door. Help her put on her coat. Stand when she comes to the table and pull out her chair for her at restaurants. Do that whether it is your mother, wife or anyone else deserving of respect. Do it with your daughter, and when grown she will reject anyone who is less than a gentleman.

16. **Tame your tongue.** I have lost track of the times I have said in public when I hear someone cursing in front of me and my children, "Hey, this is a G-rated aisle, okay?" You should not be cursing, period, or letting any corrupt communication proceed from your mouth (Ephesians 4:29), but especially keep your cool in public. Little ears are listening and learning.

17. **Respect your elders.** In the South we say, "Yes, sir," "No, ma'am," etc. We let senior citizens go first in food lines (before children) and we listen when they talk. Maybe you have other traditions where you live. Find out what they are and practice them!

18. **If you work in public, act like you want to be there.** If you work in retail, the answer to "Do you have any of these in stock in the back?" is never "Uh, naw, I think everything we got is out here already." I can hardly contain myself when I get this answer. At least go check for that customer

who is paying your paycheck! Bottom line: If you have a job working with people, act like you want to be there, whether it is pizza delivery or pastoring.

19. **Remember people's names.** Make notes if you have to, because people love to be remembered. Brownie points for remembering spouses' and kids' names!

20. **Discipline your kids.** Do not let your kids rule your own house, much less someone else's. When you visit a friend's house with them, make sure your children know they are to respect the belongings of others, as well as the people themselves. Do not enter a friend's home and start rearranging things on lower shelves. Teach your children the word *no* and, more importantly, the gravity of making a friend sad. Have a plan before entering the home of how you will discipline your child should things not go as hoped, and stick to it. We would discreetly take our child to another room and, yes, spank him or her. No open displays of shame, but private correction. This was done in love and based on Proverbs 29:15, "The rod and reproof give wisdom, but a child left to himself brings shame to his mother." And also Proverbs 22:15 (NASB): "Foolishness is bound up in the heart of a child; the rod of discipline will remove it far from him." There are plenty of other verses about discipline, period, but you cannot dodge the ones that call for spanking. Be consistent with your children, especially when in public or at a friend's home. They will think more of you, not less. Never discipline in anger, and always end by affirming your child and showing love. If you do respond in anger, always ask your child's forgiveness. God expects your child

> Imagine a society in which everyone respects one another. That begins when children are young and taught to obey you and respect others in the homes you visit as a family.

to respect you, but He also expects you to respect your child. Imagine a society in which everyone respects one another. That begins when children are young and taught to obey you and respect others in the homes you visit as a family.

So now you have my top twenty common courtesies list. Emotionally healthy people have a heart, mind their manners and are courteous at all costs!

"Finally, be ye all of one mind, having compassion one of another, love as brethren, be pitiful, be courteous" (1 Peter 3:8 KJV).

Healthy Habit Helpers

1. Name some ways you know you can be more courteous to those around you (name names if you must):

_____

_____

_____

_____

_____

Now put your hand on your heart and pray this aloud with me:

Dear God, I do want to have Your heart for others. I believe it will show if I do. Make me more tender, attentive, gentle, respectful and others minded. In Jesus' name I pray, Amen.

4

Put On a Happy Face

"On cloud nine." "Over the moon." "On top of the world." "Walking on air." "In seventh heaven." Ever noticed how most of the idioms for happiness have to do with the heavens? That is because happiness is a heavenly gift! So what *is* happiness, anyway? First, a definition: Happiness is, according to *Merriam-Webster's*, a "state of well-being characterized by emotions ranging from contentment to intense joy." While we are at it, let's also look at joy: "the emotion of great delight or happiness caused by something exceptionally good or satisfying; keen pleasure; the expression or display of glad feeling."

We often think happiness and joy are the same thing, but they are not. They are related, but not twins, sort of how a smile is different from a laugh but can originate from the same emotional source. Psalm 68:3 (NIV) says, "But may the righteous be glad and rejoice before God; may they be happy and joyful." See that? Happy *and* joyful. Two different states of being. I am going to show which one comes first, what their differences are and how they manifest themselves uniquely. You have to learn to tap in to your happy!

To start, let me ask you a question that will reveal which comes first, happiness or joy: Did you know that you can have *joy in your heart* without having *happiness in your life?* You see, joy is on the inside, and happiness is on the outside. Happiness is the manifestation of joy. It is the child of joy. Joy is a fruit of God's Spirit, but maybe joy has some fruit of its own. I believe *that* fruit is called "happiness."

If you are a Christian, you already know that the joy of the Lord is your strength (Nehemiah 8:10). You also already know that joy is one of the nine fruits of God's Spirit (Galatians 5:22–23). You probably also know that Psalm 16:11 says that in God's presence is the fullness of joy. So, if you have access to all this joy, then why does it sometimes seem invisible?

> Did you know that you can have *joy in your heart* without having *happiness in your life?*

Because joy is *supposed* to be invisible. That way, it is hidden and protected! It is constant. It is not dependent on circumstances or results. The world does not give it to you, and the world cannot take it away.

Conversely, happiness is *not* invisible. Everyone can see whether or not you are happy. You yourself know if you are unhappy, even if you are a Christian and know you are supposed to have boundless joy. You *do* have boundless joy. It is in there! You just need to know how to quickly convert it into happiness each and every day. Learn to tap in to your happy.

The secret to this quick conversion is called *gladness*. Yes, *gladness* or *glad* means everything you can imagine that involves pleasure and other happy emotions, but one dictionary actually defines *glad* like this: "contented; causing happiness or contentment, very willing. (Example: *I will be glad to help*.)."

Did you notice that glad is not joy by definition? Gladness is contentedness. Gladness *causes* happiness. Gladness is willing. *Very* willing.

129

My grandmother's name was Gladys, which means many things, including "glad" or "gladness." And she was always willing. In that sense, then, she was always "glad." If I said, "My grandmother was a glad person," you might picture a chipper, giddy, bubbly woman. That is not what *glad* means, however, and that is not how I or her children or grandchildren would describe her. But Gladys Rooks *was* willing. And contented. There was nothing too hard for her, and, trust me, she lived through plenty of hard. She birthed five babies during the Great Depression and World War II, and then, along with my granddaddy Dalton, she raised them on a thriving working farm in the Deep South. If you showed up at her door unexpectedly, she was *willing* to make you a meal. If you needed a place to sleep, she was *willing* to give you a bed. And if you needed her to "take you to town" because you were a kid spending your summer vacation on their remote farm and were bored out of your skull, well, she was willing to do that, too. Gladys was glad. She was contented. She was willing. Being glad to be willing is the secret to accessing your joy and converting it into happiness. God wants you to "be glad" so that you can then be happy and joyful!

Now listen again to Psalm 68:3: "But may the righteous *be glad* and rejoice before God; may they be happy and joyful" (emphasis mine). Gladness precedes happiness and joy, and the command is to make yourself *be glad*. Come on, face it— sometimes, when circumstances do not go the way you need or want, you are not willing to be happy. You think if you act unhappy enough that God will notice and zap something for you. You want your situation to change before you act happy. And then you wonder where your joy went! God is saying to you, *Be willing. Be glad.* Gladness is your bridge from joy to happiness. And just listen what joy and gladness can do together:

Gladness and joy will overtake them, and sorrow and sighing will flee away.

> Isaiah 35:10 NIV

They shall obtain *gladness and joy*; and sorrow and mourning shall flee away.

> Isaiah 51:11 KJV

May those who delight in my vindication shout for *joy and gladness.*

> Psalm 35:27 NIV

They are led in with *joy and gladness*; they enter the palace of the king.

> Psalm 45:15 NIV

When gladness and joy get together, it changes your countenance. You look happier. This is important because if you are walking around looking like you have been baptized in lemon juice, something is wrong. You can *see* the fruit of gladness and joy, and it is happiness. But God does not stop there. Did you know that joy and gladness have a *sound*? "Let me *hear* joy and gladness" (Psalm 51:8 NIV).

Hear joy and gladness? How do you do that? What does joy and gladness sound like? "Joy and gladness will be found in her, thanksgiving and the sound of singing" (Isaiah 51:3). There is that word again; *sound.* And Jeremiah talks four times about the sounds of joy and gladness (Jeremiah 7:34; 25:10; 33:11; 48:33 NIV).

It is evident that when joy and gladness get together, they make some noise. But what is the sound of joy and gladness? Laughter! (In the next healthy living habit, we will explore the marvel medicine of laughter and how it actually brings health to the body and peace to your mind.)

In January 2005, *Time* magazine featured an issue entitled "The Science of Happiness." Eastgate was in its first month as a church when it was released, and I used the many articles of this issue and dozens of Scriptures to preach my first sermon there. One piece inside explored questions like "What are your major sources of happiness?" and shared the results of a poll in which this question was asked. The number-one answer (77 percent) was "Relationships with your children." Almost as many, 76 percent, said "Friendships." Other

What are your major sources of happiness? answers earning percentages in the 60s and 70s were "Contributing to the lives of others," "Spouse," "The degree of control over your life and destiny," "Relationship with parents," and "Religious, spiritual life and worship." Trailing somewhat behind, at 50 percent, was "Holidays."[1]

And what about money? Actually, money ranked fourteenth on the *Time* poll of what makes people happy. The article mentioned the Great Depression and the hardships that came during the late 1920s through the early 1940s, when money was tight for most families, and yet cited that "depression" is more typical of today's society, in which people have more money than ever before. In fact, depression is considered an epidemic and is three to ten times more common now than two generations ago. It seems we went from the Great Depression to a greater depression. So, no, money does not make you happier.

Recap:

Joy is on the inside, but happiness is where? *On the outside.* And what must you do when you do not feel happy? *Be willing to (glad).*

1. "Feeling Good in the U.S." (*Time* poll conducted December 13–14, 2004), *Time*, January 17, 2005, A5.

And what do joy and gladness look like? *Happiness.*

And what do joy and gladness sound like? *Laughter!*

Emotionally healthy people understand the importance of gladness as a bridge between joy and happiness, and they also have revelation of the power of a good laugh. Are you ready to study the miracle of laughter? You are going to love it!

"So I concluded there is nothing better than to be happy and enjoy ourselves as long as we can" (Ecclesiastes 3:12 NLT).

Healthy Habit Helpers

1. Name some things that "zap your happy" and the ways you can "tap in to your happy" when you encounter them:

_____

_____

_____

Now put your hand on your heart and pray this aloud with me:

Father, I want to be happier and I want to make others around me happy. Most of all, I want to make You happy. I give You my attitude, countenance and words for a Holy Ghost happiness makeover. I am glad (willing) to submit to Your changes. In Jesus' name, Amen.

5

Laugh Out Loud

You have heard that laughter is the best medicine, but do you believe it? When is the last time you had a head-raising, side-splitting laugh-out-loud moment? I mean, if you knew there was really such a thing as "the best medicine" on the planet, you would want to stock up and down it daily, right? Hourly! Science and Scripture agree that laughter is a necessary component to the emotionally healthy person's life. It can heal, slow aging, control pain, relieve stress and enhance pleasure. Smiling does not, whether it is a "Pan American smile"—a polite but not heartfelt expression that involves mouth muscles and little else—or a full-blown Duchenne smile, in which the muscles around the eyes contract involuntarily, expressing a sincere joy. "I will forget my complaint, I will change my expression, and smile" (Job 9:27 NIV).

Laughter is a different phenomenon altogether. It is like exercise! That is why your stomach sometimes feels sore after a good belly laugh. Your neck, abs, diaphragm, respiratory system and facial muscles all get a complete workout. Some people even use their hands, arms, legs and back muscles when laughing (present company included). It benefits digestive functions, as well. Robust laughter, it is estimated, can burn calories equal to several minutes on an exercise bike or rowing machine. It also gives the voice box a workout, since the number-one difference between a smile and a laugh is . . . sound! Even the definition of the word *laughter* includes "to express amusement or satisfaction with inarticulate sounds."

Researchers have discovered an amazing number of ways that laughter promotes health. For starters, it can protect your heart: According to a study at the University of Maryland Medical Center, laughter, along with a healthy sense of humor, may help protect against a heart attack and heart disease. The study revealed that people with heart disease were 40 percent less likely to laugh at various circumstances compared to people of the same age without heart disease.[1] Laughter does, after all, quite a lot to exercise your heart. During the two stages of laughter—the arousal phase, when the heart rate increases, and the resolution phase, when the heart rests—the heart rate reaches up to 120 beats per minute, and laughing can lower your blood pressure, increase vascular flow, raise your pulse and boost the immune system.

Humor literally changes your biochemical state.

As far back as biblical days, mankind understood the therapeutic value of humor. But it was not until Norman Cousins's 1979 *Anatomy of an Illness*[2] that the general public and scientists began taking a serious look at the potential value of therapeutic laughter, humor and play. In the 1960s, Cousins,

1. "Laughter Is Good Medicine for Your Heart, According to a New UMMC Study," University of Maryland Medical Center, November 15, 2000, http://umm .edu/news-and-events/news-releases/2000/laughter-is-good-for-your-heart-accord ing-to-a-new-ummc-study.
2. Norman Cousins, *Anatomy of an Illness: As Perceived by the Patient* (New York: W. W. Norton, 1979).

then editor of the *Saturday Review*, had returned from a visit to Moscow to become suddenly ill and was hospitalized with a high fever, severe pain and decreasing mobility. His doctors were confounded, and Cousins made a bold decision to leave the hospital and try a different treatment: He checked into a hotel and watched some of his favorite comedy movies and television shows. In short, he intentionally used laughter as medicine. The pain eventually and entirely disappeared. Cousins wrote his book about the experience in 1979, and people around the world took notice. The result has been psychoneuroimmunology, or humor therapy. In this field of medicine, only laughter is used as medication. It led to the development in 1992 of a United States Office of Alternative Medicine, officially granting legitimacy to the old proverb that "laughter is the best medicine."

Researchers have described two main types of humor: "Passive humor" happens when observing a comedy routine, film or even a funny commercial. "Humor production" involves choosing humor and optimism in stressful situations. It is thought that being able to keep a positive attitude and laugh at oneself and at life's sometimes-stressful events can be very health giving.

Humor has been seen as medicinal throughout recorded history. The Bible lends proof of this in Proverbs 17:22, "A joyful heart is good medicine." Even as far back as the thirteenth century, some surgeons used humor to distract patients from the pain of surgery. Because laughing stimulates the cardiovascular system, respiratory system, circulatory system, muscular system and more, it should be no surprise that it is a powerful tool during recovery, as well. Many hospitals are incorporating special rooms stocked with funny movies, books, games and sometimes even comedians or clowns to help make people laugh and heal faster. Evidently, laughing out loud is more healing than mere intellectual amusement. The Cancer Treatment Centers of America actually offer humor therapy sessions (also called humor groups or Laughter Clubs) as a tool for cancer patients and their families to find relief and healing.[3]

You already know that stress can kill. We are going to discuss that more in the next healthy living habit, but while we are on the topic of laughter, let's look at its mental and emotional benefits. If you have been paying attention in your own life, you already have a hunch that these facts are true, and now you will understand the science behind your hunch:

1. Laughter stimulates the release of certain neurotransmitters that enhance pleasure, calm nerves, etc. It helps create opioids, which are natural substances produced by our bodies that mimic opiates like morphine and codeine. When manufactured in pill form, opiates are highly addictive and emotionally numbing. Laughter is much safer, and free.

2. Laughter releases endorphins in the brain, our bodies' natural painkillers. It causes a bodily chemical change and interrupts the pain cycle of illness, whether physical or psychological.

3. The same chemicals are released whether you react to something funny or manufacture a "fake" laugh. Your body does not know the difference, so force a fake laugh in private when in need of a boost!

4. Hearty laughter stimulates the right and left sides of the brain by increasing oxygen flow to the brain. With more oxygen, we have higher levels of mental processing, more creativity and increased ability to problem solve.

5. Laughter slows the processes of aging by influencing central nervous system connections to the lymph nodes and multiple hormonal secretions (increasing good ones and decreasing the bad).

3. "Laughter Therapy," Cancer Treatment Centers of America, accessed April 21, 2017, http://www.cancercenter.com/treatments/laughter-therapy/.

As Mark Twain once said, "The human race has only one really effective weapon, and that's laughter."

Unfortunately, since humor does not require a costly, patented pill that can financially benefit a pharmaceutical company, there is no real source of funding for studies of long-term benefits of humor therapy (despite thousands of years of documented testimonies). But we know from experience that laughter is good medicine. It is contagious—otherwise, why would television producers plant "laughers" in studio audiences? Thankfully, there is no such thing as "humor toxicity" or "laughter overdose," and perhaps we can even say "a laugh a day keeps the doctor away." "The One enthroned in heaven laughs" (Psalm 2:4 NIV).

A laugh a day keeps the doctor away.

Maybe you grew up in humorless environments in which fun was deemphasized. If so, laughing out loud might feel awkward. But surely you want to live longer, control pain and relieve stress, right? Then incorporate these fifteen tips into your life so you can become an emotionally healthy person:

- Attempt every day to laugh at situations and stay positive.
- Laugh (out loud to yourself) when tense; feel yourself relax.
- Imagine previous funny situations to replace the situation you are in.
- Remember that your smile and laugh can help someone else's tension.
- Put time, focus and energy into experiences that make you laugh.
- Start welcoming silly stuff to interrupt your day.
- Observe young children and babies to learn the art of delight.
- Increase your exposure to comedy: movies, sitcoms, games, etc.

- Hang around funny people, or, better yet, marry a funny person.
- Take a five- to ten-minute humor break every day.
- Read jokes and try them out on friends! Laugh at your poor delivery.
- Avoid conversations or relationships with negative people.
- Avoid news that frightens or distresses you and makes you sad.
- Pray for God to fill you with the joy of the Lord. It is your strength!
- Ask someone to tickle you. (Couldn't resist, sorry.)

In the nineteenth century, malignancy and depression became synonymous.[4] Nearly two thousand years ago, the physician Galen noted that cheerful women were less likely to get cancer than women who were depressed. Proverbs 31:25 (NIV) says, "She is clothed with strength and dignity; she can laugh at the days to come." Friends, laughter is a miraculous psychological and physiological phenomenon that works like medicine. Whereas most drugs affect everyone differently, laughter always remains the same.

"Our mouths were filled with laughter" . . . (Psalm 126:2 NIV).

Healthy Habit Helpers

1. Name three ways you can fit more laughter and positivity into your life:

_____

_____

4. Marianna Karamanou, Elias Tzavellas, Konstantinos Laios, Michalis Koutsilieris, and George Androutsos, "Melancholy as a Risk Factor for Cancer: A Historical Overview," *JBUON* 21, no. 3 (2016), https://www.jbuon.com/pdfs/JBUON-21-3-34.pdf.

_____

_____

Now put your hand on your heart and pray this aloud with me:

Okay, God, life is tense sometimes. I need Your help to stay positive and laugh, even if it means laughing at myself. Help me never to lose my laugh, and help me to be a source of joy and laughter to others. In Jesus' name, Amen!

6

De-stress Your Distress

The world is distressed. Undoubtedly, we are experiencing a stress epidemic, and indirectly stress is most likely our number-one killer. Physiologically speaking, there are two kinds of stress: distress, which is the negative kind of stress; and eustress, a positive kind of stress. While distress increases stress hormones such as cortisol, growth hormone, beta-endorphin, corticotrophin, prolactin and others, eustress decreases those hormones and increases the activity of natural killer cells that help fight disease. (In this healthy living habit, I will be using the word *stress* to refer to distress.)

Stress wears down our immune systems, resulting in greater risk of sickness and disease. Our generation is treating the disease instead of the cause. Instead of seeking God for resolutions to stressors like toxic relationships, financial debt, internal sadness, electronic overstimulation, etc., many turn to pills to help balance the emotional storm inside.

To be precise, 94,836,220 Americans make this choice. That is right, almost 30 percent of Americans are on some type of psychiatric drug.[1] That includes more than 41 million on anti-depressants, more than 36 million on anti-anxiety meds, more than 10 million on ADHD drugs and more than 6 million on antipsychotics. That means almost 30 percent of your neighborhood. Maybe even 30 percent of your church. Close to 1 out of every 3 people you know. Many websites put that figure at closer to 1 in 6, but I got mine from the 2013 Vector One National (VONA) and Total Patient Tracker databases from IMS Health. VONA is recognized by the FDA and is unique and unbiased because it measures retail dispensing of prescriptions, or the frequency with which drugs move out of retail pharmacies into the

Stress wears down our immune systems, resulting in greater risk of sickness and disease. Our generation is treating the disease instead of the cause.

hands of consumers. Since 2002, the Vector One database has documented information on more than 8 billion prescriptions from 200 million unique patients.[2] Their near–95 million total for Americans on psychiatric drugs is staggering, but likely accurate.

Some say "shame on the shrinks." Others say, "thank God for these meds!" Let me just say that I have seen lives saved by people getting on antidepressants or anxiety medications. I have also seen others ruined on them due to addiction. The best success I have observed has come to those who, confronted with evidence they could not live or function without psychiatric

1. "Total Number of People Taking Psychiatric Drugs in the United States," Citizen's Commission on Human Rights International, https://www.cchrint.org/psychiatric-drugs/people-taking-psychiatric-drugs/. The site's breakdown of the individuals on each class of drug totals this astronomically high number.

2. Claudia Karwoski, Pharm.D., Memorandum to the Drug Safety and Risk Management and the Dermatologic and Ophthalmic Drugs Advisory Committees, FDA Center for Drug Evaluation and Research, November 15, 2011, https://www.fda.gov/downloads/AdvisoryCommittees/CommitteesMeetingMaterials/Drugs/DermatologicandOphthalmicDrugsAdvisoryCommittee/UCM281375.pdf.

pharmaceutical intervention, took the drugs for a brief period and then weaned off of them with the help of integrative remedies to stabilize chemical imbalances, adding in Christian counseling and persistent prayer for extra support. These drugs were created to be used for brief periods and would be ideal if used as such, but, according to a study published in the *British Journal of Psychology*, patients are staying on antidepressants 50 percent longer than they did in the 1990s.[3] The average duration a person is on these types of drugs is now nearly six months (169 days), compared to just under four months (112 days) in the mid-'90s. On average, one in four patients take the pills for an average of fifteen months, as opposed to eight months twenty years ago. But many are staying on them for decades. The real crisis for these "decaders" is that one often plateaus on such medications and must switch to another, but no new antidepressants are due to be released in the next decade.

> The main reason . . . is that the NHS and healthcare providers in other countries do not want to pay the bill for new drugs that will have to go through expensive trials. . . . "We are not going to get any more new drugs for depression in the next decade simply because the pharmaceutical industry is not investing in research," said Goodwin. "It can't make money on these drugs."[4]

Those issues, coupled with one of the medications not working at all for many, create a need for alternative answers to their stress and mental and neurological illnesses.

It was this plight and my own that set me on a quest. As I shared previously, I used to suffer violent convulsions, not to

3. Sarah Knapton, "Patients on Antidepressants for 50 Percent Longer than in 1990s," *Telegraph*, January 15, 2017, http://www.telegraph.co.uk/science/2017/01/15/patients-antidepressants-50-per-cent-longer-1990s/.
4. Sarah Boseley, "No New Antidepressants Likely in Next Decade, Say Scientists," *Guardian*, January 11, 2017, https://www.theguardian.com/science/2017/jan/11/no-new-antidepressants-likely-next-decade-say-scientists.

mention decades' worth of smaller absence seizures. Neurologists could never explain why the antiseizure medications would not provide full seizure coverage for me. Much of it I attributed to undeniable spiritual warfare involving what Mark 9 calls a "deaf and dumb spirit." But it turns out there was also a molecular explanation. Remember that God is a triune God, and so for every Goliath you face, He will give you a physical strategy, a spiritual strategy and an emotional strategy. The result? A physical victory, a spiritual victory and an emotional victory. Wholeness!

> Remember: God is a triune God, and so for every Goliath you face, He will give you a physical strategy, a spiritual strategy and an emotional strategy.

So what was the physical explanation for why doctors could not achieve full success for me on seizure medicines? It was the same reason that many psychiatric drugs do not work for sufferers: something called the blood-brain barrier (BBB). This barrier is our brain's miraculous security system. If there were no barrier, all sorts of foods, chemicals and toxins we encounter might very well seep into the brain. The downside of this is that many medications will not cross it. "The blood-brain barrier," writes Dr. William Pardridge in *Neuro Rx*: The Journal for the American Society of Experimental NeuroTherapeutics*, "is formed by the brain capillary endothelium and excludes from the brain 100% of large-molecule neurotherapeutics and more than 98% of all small-molecule drugs."[5]

Did you catch that? An estimated *98 percent* of all medications for brain/mind disorders are unable to infiltrate the BBB, and 100 percent of today's treatments are unable to aid the

5. William M. Pardridge, "The Blood-Brain Barrier: Bottleneck in Brain Drug Development," *NeuroRx*: The Journal of the American Society for Experimental NeuroTherapeutics* 2, no. 1 (2005), https://www.ncbi.nlm.nih.gov/pmc/articles/PMC539316/pdf/neurorx002000003.pdf.

brain at all if their molecular compounds are too large. Imagine the implications: millions upon millions of suffering patients who take daily medicine but find no consistent relief from their neurological ailments. And for many who do, the relief comes at the high price of countless side effects, including multiple neurological malfunctions and manifestations.

So if 100 percent of large-molecule neurotherapeutic drugs and 98 percent of small-molecule ones are not penetrating the BBB, what can? David Stewart has the answer. He has a Ph.D. and is a registered aromatherapist and author of *Healing Oils of the Bible* (Care Publishing, 2003). In one of his many articles on the healing properties of oil, "The Blood-Brain Barrier," he writes,

> The American Medical Association has said that if they could find an agent that would pass the blood-brain barrier, they would be able to find cures for ailments such as Lou Gehrig's disease, multiple sclerosis, Alzheimer's disease, and Parkinson's disease. Such agents already exist and have been available since Biblical times. The agents, of course, are essential oils—particularly those containing the brain oxygenating molecules of sesquiterpenes.[6]

Even having personally experimented for ten years with essential oils, I never knew that some could pass through the BBB while others could not. That explained why certain oils I tried had little to no effect on my condition (be it a headache, stress or a seizure): because they had a very low sesquiterpene count, and only sesquiterpenes have molecules tiny enough to pass through the BBB. It is their molecular "tininess" that makes sesquiterpenes so aromatic (and costly), since the smaller the molecule, the easier it passes when inhaled through the nasal

6. David Stewart, Ph.D., R.A., "The Blood-Brain Barrier," *Raindrop Messenger*, January 2003, http://www.raindroptraining.com/messenger/v1n1.html#one.

passages directly into the limbic areas of the brain, not to mention through the BBB when applied topically.

Armed with this new knowledge, in the summer of 2016 I set out to pinpoint which essential oils best calmed the brain and then choose from among them only those from the sesquiterpene family. That way, these miraculous brain-nourishing oils could actually pass through the BBB and accomplish their goal, which was to quiet my electrically malfunctioning brain. Thus, Quiet Brain® Essential Oil Blend was born.

Combining only pure therapeutic-grade versions of oils like frankincense, myrrh, lavender and more, the first bottle (and every bottle since) was created in an environment of worship and silence. I listened for and documented the precise recipe, and I felt led not to dilute it with any carrier oil, resulting in a very potent blend. Afterward, my husband and I prayed for God to transform Quiet Brain into anointing oil. And then the instruction came by the Holy Spirit: *Register it with the United States Patent and Trademark Office and conduct a case study.* So, after researching what the FDA considered to be a case study, and complying with those standards, we started our first small trial conducted on family, friends and congregants who had diagnosed neurological issues. The results stunned us all over the coming weeks: relief from PTSD; ending migraine in less than five minutes when given at onset; relief of essential tremor; halting convulsions upon application; alleviating anxieties, depressions, insomnia, stress, ADHD and more. The testimonies have continued to pour in from all over the world, and Quiet Brain is now one of the most ordered items in my online store.[7] These dramatic results also led us to seek the legal protection of a United States patent for the proprietary recipe. Each bottle is a

7. You can read more testimonies and order Quiet Brain at www.QuietBrainOil.com.

ten-week supply, and many say they feel it working from the very first application. *How can that not be supernatural?* It is naturally supernatural.

Now, listen, in my Shop At Home Network days, I was briefed by our legal department to never say on air, "Your results may vary," but, instead, "Your results *will* vary." So I tell you that here, too: Your results *will* vary. We make no medical claims and only give client testimonies so you can see what the oil is doing for some. It is composed entirely of ingredients made by God on the third day of creation—oils pressed from grasses, trees, flowers, etc.—and so I know God is *in* the oil. But I also think He is *on* it, since each batch is prayed over by pastors and will be for as long as it is in production. I believe Quiet Brain is more like an anointing oil than a medicinal oil, as evidenced by the dramatic testimonials. We believe firmly that this is a viable option in the war on your sleep, nerves, brain and peace.

> Afterward, my husband and I prayed for God to transform Quiet Brain into anointing oil.

I am happy to say that my own brain is neurologically quieter than it has ever been, and yet my creativity has not dulled, nor has my focus. Quiet Brain calms but does not sedate. That is good news for this busy mom, wife, daughter, pastor, author, nutritionist and friend. Oh . . . and inventor!

Healthy Habit Helpers

1. Name your major life stresses and what you proactively do to calm them:

   _____

   _____

   _____

Now put your hand on your heart and pray this aloud with me:

Dear God: Aaaaaah! I need You every busy second of every busy day! Right now I fling every care and distress I have upon You. Take it! Now give me peace in my heart and a strategy for my body and mind. In Jesus' name I pray, Amen.

7

Never Be Discouraged Again

Almost twenty years ago, I made the decision never to be discouraged again. I had become altogether weary of waiting on God for many things at once. Sickness has always been the enemy's weapon of choice against me since I was very young (even though he always saw God glorified through healing or patience), and in that season Satan had pulled out all of his big guns against my body. I had almost lost my life many dozens of times, and I lived with constant bruises, headaches and a torn tongue. That trial alone would cause most people to stay in bed with the covers pulled over their heads (impossible with the five kids I had at the time), but the combination of that and a severe financial crisis tried to drag me into an invisible pit of despair. Our family's choice to support Chris in walking away from a very comfortable life in the corporate music industry to pursue more ministry had left us wondering whether we had even heard God or not. He had spoken so clearly! We had obeyed to the letter! So here we were, about to lose our house, car, credit, and . . . minds. Oh, yeah, and my life.

We needed healing and finances. "Health and wealth." We referred to them as our "faith twins." We allowed God to conceive in us something too big to birth on our own, which was total physical freedom for me from all convulsions and financial freedom for Chris, allowing him (us) to be in full-time ministry. But the enemy opposed us at every turn. He wanted us to miss Egypt's meat and go back. We chose to stay, of course, but in the darkest of days, when doubt would come calling (along with a creditor or a symptom), we had to make the choice each time to stand. We became increasingly efficient at dismissing doubt and choosing faith. We no longer squandered energy on "Why me, God?" or "Did I not hear You?" or "What will others think?" Complaining became a thing of the past. It wasted time. It degenerated focus and atrophied faith. You learn these things as you go along and decide that if you cannot control the circumstances, you can at least control yourself. So we did.

It was at that juncture that I decided to start viewing discouragement as sin.

It was at that juncture that I decided to start viewing discouragement as sin. Same with fear. If I could just equate them to sin, then I knew I would steer clear, and it has worked for these near twenty years. Besides, Romans 14:23 says, "For whatever does not proceed from faith is sin," so, since discouragement does not proceed from faith, that is scriptural-enough proof for me that discouragement is sin.

Now when discouragement comes calling (i.e., circumstances that evoke emotional disappointment), I employ these three steps and never (ever) experience a hiccup in my day or mood:

1. While the emotion is fresh and alive, I find some space to be alone in prayer, and I spend every drop of that emotion in prayer. This self-discipline is to prayer what motor oil is to engine care. *Do not waste* even a dribble of that

emotion. Listen to me: Do not call a friend first and vent. Do not complain to your spouse (process for prayer but no complaining). Do not pass "Go" . . . go directly to your knees and talk it out with God! And do not complain or vent there, either. In fact, if you already know God's will on the matter (if He has already made it clear in His Word or through a prior word of direction), then just skip the prayer and start thanking Him for the answer that you are sure is on its way. Then, spend the rest of the time reminding the enemy of his nearing defeat. You will know instinctively when it is time to get up and move on. You will feel the divine exchange occur: your mood for His peace.

2. Get busy serving. My friend, Sue, used to always dream about tennis, and we could never figure out why. Finally, one day I asked, "Sue, who starts these tennis games in your dreams?" She said, "Hmmm . . . I do. Why?" I said, "God is saying you are supposed to be *serving*!" Sure enough, Sue is always happiest when she is serving. I have never seen anything like it! She could be dog tired, running on empty, sleep deprived and hangry (hungry + angry), and yet when she is serving somewhere—to a shut-in, with children, at church, etc.—she is all smiles. I think we all love to feel needed, and serving accomplishes that. So after you are done praying (number 1), get up and get serving.

3. After you have prayed and served, do something fun to reward yourself. The quickest, cheapest thing I do is watch a funny movie. Everybody has his or her "go-to" flicks that bring a smile. Watch one. Fix a healthy snack. Invite someone to join you. Just change the mood in your house. You "fixed" the solution in prayer and sealed it with service; now change the atmosphere in your home. If you

do not have time for a movie, music is just as powerful. I usually play a mix of worship music coupled with fun tunes from my teen years.

Granted, you do not always have time to pray, serve and watch a movie after every discouragement! But remember spiritual Healthy Living Habit No. 8: "Accept No Substitutes." Emotionally healthy people go to God first. There is always time to pray. God works within your time constraints, and, besides, it takes all of ten seconds to move from bad news to bowing your head to entrusting it to God to thanking Him and gloating at your enemy. Seriously!

I feel very sorry for people who never make the discouragement-sin connection. Discouragement is like a big cushy chair, and some people like to climb in it when things get hard. They behave like there is no other chair in the room, and they certainly never consider that what they really need to do is just stand. I am so glad I did. The little ears in my home that were listening to me back then grew up and became adults who now know how to resist fear and discouragement. *Who is listening to you?*

One of the other ways I change my mood (number 3) is to write poetry. It is cheaper than therapy and wraps everything up in a nice, tidy bow. I wrote this poem during one of my last moments of discouragement, almost twenty years ago. This gal *knew* that health and wealth (and full-time ministry) were in her future. She was right!

The Wait

I've got a problem; maybe you have the same
Mine searches me out, and it knows me by name
Its goal is to use me and leave me ashamed
to kill, steal and destroy

It met no resistance, once upon a time
For years I allowed it, for years I was blind
And then I awoke and saw what was mine
although I have still yet to hold it

I've asked believing; I've fasted; I've prayed
I've heard God's instruction and learned to obey
I've seen others get what I want in one day
and learned to love without envy

I spoke to the mountain; I've named and I've claimed
I've bound and I've loosed and had things stay the same
I've warred with the Name that's above all names
while it seemed to profit me nothing

Through visions and dreams my instruction's been sealed
Hearing more than can ever be shared or revealed
Staying quiet so God's secret plans are concealed
and released then at just the right moment

I've trusted, rested, hoped for and doubted
I've ached with self-pity, I've grieved and I've pouted
I've seen power come when I whispered or shouted
for I've learned it's not your volume, but your authority

I've seen my protection in prayer as I kneeled
I've seen with my eyes His great buckler and shield
discovering wholeness as you wait to be healed
And I have dwelled in the shelter of the Most High

I've drank from a fountain, in gulps and in sips
I've seen the Son shine in a total eclipse
I've tasted sweet praise pouring over bruised lips
and I've felt Him inhabit that praise

Hungry for more, I've tasted some power
I've drank from a cup that is sweet, and still sour
I've starved my flesh hoping to feast at some hour
only to feast once again on the fruit of patience

I swam upstream in water that's muddy
I've knocked and I've knocked 'til my knuckles are bloody
I've heard people say without words that I'm nutty
and can honestly say I've died to all reputation

Blessed is he who does not see, yet believes
Perhaps it's an office we all should achieve
The price though, is more than we ever perceive
when we start praying those dangerous prayers for
    patience

Does faith say this is the day, if it's not?
Can God stretch a scene if He's building a plot?
Do you judge those who wait, or want what they've got?
Knowing that it's through faith & patience we receive
    God's promises

We can't live without it, we can barely live through it
It's a fruit of God's Spirit, and there's no shortcut to it
If you find one, it only reveals that you blew it
'Cause King James said it best when he called it
    "longsuffering."

Are you willing to wait? Are you able to learn?
Is getting an answer your only concern?
Can anything hide your impatience that burns
from a God who knows your heart and is a consuming fire?

Those who wait on the Lord, they will find great strength
Strength that cannot be owned by the proud, but the meek
It's the joy of the Lord, without which you're weak
Strength by which you can run against a troop and defeat
    your enemies

Your waiting is precious; your trials are gold;
Your tears liquid praise when the battle gets old;
Though the waters rise and the rivers overflow
You're winning! You're winning! You're winning!

© Laura Harris Smith

154

"Cast your burden on the LORD, and he will sustain you; he will never permit the righteous to be moved" (Psalm 55:22).

Healthy Habit Helpers

1. Name your major temptations for discouragement and what you are going to do the next time they come:

_____

_____

_____

Now put your hand on your heart and pray this aloud with me:

Dear God, You have my complete trust. I need not fear or sigh. I thank You in advance for how You are answering my prayers! And also . . .

Dear Discouragement: It's over. We're finished. I am trading you for prayer, serving and peace. Thank You, God, for this revelation! In Jesus' name I pray, Amen.

8

Pick Your Battles

In Healthy Living Habit No. 5 for the spirit, "Do the Honors," we discussed at length what defines, precedes and follows a lifestyle of honor. We also contemplated the difficulty in showing honor to one who honors none. We are not to sow honor into the dishonorable by supporting celebrities, public figures or leaders who lead dishonorable lives.

So, then, what do you do when the dishonorable leader you disdain is actually your president, governor, mayor or other elected official? What if he or she is your professor, pastor, sports coach, spouse or boss? What do you do if you do not see that person showing respect to others? Are you expected to respect him or her regardless? Or do you treat the person as you would a dishonorable celebrity, from whom you should just withdraw your support? Yes, there is a measure of honor that is due each leader in your life, community or nation—*but* let's walk this through for each of these relationships. Emotionally healthy people know how to pick their battles. They must learn which relationships and situations call for war, which ones call for withdrawal and which ones call for waiting.

Romans 13:1–7 (NIV, emphasis mine) will be our text for this healthy living habit.

> Let every person *be subject to the governing authorities.* For there is no authority except from God, and *those that exist have been instituted by God.* Therefore *whoever resists the authorities resists what God has appointed, and those who resist will incur judgment.* For rulers are not a terror to good conduct, but to bad. *Would you have no fear of the one who is in authority? Then do what is good, and you will receive his approval,* for he is God's servant for your good. But if you do wrong, be afraid, for he does not bear the sword in vain. For he is the servant of God, an avenger who carries out God's wrath on the wrongdoer. *Therefore one must be in subjection, not only to avoid God's wrath but also for the sake of conscience.* For the same reason you also pay taxes, for the authorities are ministers of God, attending to this very thing. *Pay to all what is owed to them: taxes to whom taxes are owed, revenue to whom revenue is owed, respect to whom respect is owed, honor to whom honor is owed.*

There is much in this passage to unpack, but the essence is that we are to submit to *all* governing authorities, give them our respect and show them honor. If we feel we cannot, or if we feel afraid to remain under their rule and wait for change, we have an option. Let's begin with elected officials.

Elected Government Officials. If you do not feel you can support certain elected officials in your national or local government, you have the option to geographically move out from their jurisdiction, but you do not have the right to cause chaos, rebel or overthrow them. Why? I believe the answer is in verse 3: "Would you have no fear of the one who is in authority? Then do what is good, and you will receive his approval." Since the entire passage outlines how to behave toward those officials *over* you, if you have already vowed within yourself that you will not

157

wait it out peacefully and pray earnestly for change and that you cannot submit to them, I would say that to "do what is good" means to come out from under them. Move. If you cannot stand your mayor, "do what is good" and find a new city. You bring judgment upon yourself if you are constantly protesting in the streets, disrupting the peace and getting arrested. If you really want to make an impact, remove your taxes and income and let them feel it in the economy, because if it is that bad, others will be going with you.

Same with all government officials. If you absolutely cannot endure your governor for some life-threatening reason (this currently does not exist in the American republic, but we know it did during the days of deadly racial injustices condoned by governing officials), then prayerfully move to another state. If you are in *immediate* mortal danger under your president, find a new one in another country, because your country is not getting another one until the next election (or the next). If I were living in a country in which an ungodly president or prime minister was harming our whole nation, and I had waited patiently and prayed but seen no changes for my family's physical safety, I would not remain under his or her heavy hand. I would *prayerfully* begin the relocation process, and I know God would make a way for my family to flee. To stick around and cause a ruckus would bring perpetual judgment upon myself legally, criminally and scripturally, accordingly to Romans 13. Make no mistake, that ungodly, dishonorable leader will have to answer to God. But so will I. He or she may not obey Scripture, but I will. And I will be blessed as a result, whereas that leader will not.

Employers. It is the same if you have a boss you cannot tolerate or submit to. You can either constantly complain, call out and gossip behind his or her back, or you can just find a new job! Remember Proverbs 27:18 (NASB): "He who cares for his master will be honored." So go find a master you can care for (and care about). And remember: You cannot be over until you learn to come under, so practice being under by showing honor to those in authority over you.

Coaches and Teachers. Same goes for your sports coach, college professor, teacher and/or club leaders. If they are so intolerable that you cannot show up with a smile, then bow out and look elsewhere. If you are out of options and there is no other team to which you can move, class to which you can transfer or club you can join, then God is obviously saying that He wants you to learn to stay and submit. He will protect you, and you will be stronger when the season or semester is over.

Pastors and Church Leaders. The previous advice is also good for your relationship with your pastor. If you feel you absolutely cannot honor your pastor (you should at least be able to honor the office), you should peacefully find another church family rather than dividing the one you have. Redistribute your respect. Always consider, though, that God may want you to stay and grow. God is into growth, big time.

Spouses, Parents and Other Family. Honor redistribution is an entirely different matter when it comes to family. Family is blood. You cannot go find a new mother, divorce your brother or fire your father. You *can* divorce your spouse, but the pain will resonate through your entire legacy for years to come, even if no children are involved. Always try to choose honor and stay. Seek counsel. Forgive. You may not like your husband or feel he is worth honoring, but maybe he does not think he can lead, and your honor will make him rise to the occasion. Treat him like the man you want him to be. Pray for him. The same advice goes to husbands who do not feel their wives are worth honoring. Whereas in all the other

159

relationships we have discussed, you have the option to relocate and redistribute your respect to other leaders, marriage is a relationship worth fighting for. So are relationships with parents and children. Those are always battles worth picking, and winning.

Like no other time in history, people seem poised and ready to pick a fight. An international generation of hundreds of millions has been told they can do anything, and they are now all trying to do it simultaneously. "Everybody wins" has backfired, creating an atmosphere of sorry losers. People are casting off restraint and rioting in the streets. The love of many is growing cold because lawlessness abounds. I saw it for myself when I went to Washington, D.C., in January 2017 for the inauguration of a new American president.

I went to D.C. because I took a vow in a vivid dream in 1999 to pray for America, and I have gone to great lengths to keep it. I have prayed on-site at national monuments, in the belly of an old American Revolutionary War ship, in airplanes, on top of skyscrapers overlooking cities and, yes, at our nation's most protested presidential inauguration to date. Chris and I went as pastors to pray and to attend the Presidential Inaugural Prayer Breakfast and other events, and while there we made a point of having deliberate conversations with both Democrats and Republicans. And I noticed something that each of the "battle pickers" had in common: None of them identified as Christian or had an intimate walk with Jesus Christ (because we were pastors, people were really opening up to us). They seemed to have no revelation that God is always in control, and so they seemed to feel the need to take matters into their own hands. I came to the conclusion that protesting must be a necessary release for these people because they do not have the venting mechanism that prayer automatically provides, nor the Comforter (the Holy Spirit) living in them to provide comfort. They might very well explode if they do not protest. Who knows, with my personality, if I did not have the Holy Spirit, I would probably be protesting every injustice that came down the pike. Thank God, I know how to vent in prayer, trust God and pick my battles. I have learned the art of warring on my knees in prayer and being patient to see God change others, including my leaders. He required my submission to them in the meantime, and I became a stealth weapon in His hand to alter the situation from the inside. So do you see the benefits of waiting now? You gain tremendous advantage in waiting and watching, including attracting the favor and protection of God for obeying His Word. I think if more of us would wait in prayer and let God show us how He is working behind the scenes, we would learn the art of withdrawal or waiting and run less quickly into war.

> This is what the LORD says to you: "Do not be afraid or discouraged because of this vast army. For the battle is not yours, but God's. . . . You will not have to fight this battle. Take up your positions; stand firm and see the deliverance the LORD will give you. . . . Do not be afraid; do not be discouraged."
>
> 2 Chronicles 20:15, 17 NIV

> And that all this assembly may know that the LORD saves not with sword and spear. For the battle is the LORD's, and he will give you into our hand.
>
> 1 Samuel 17:47

> And Moses said to the people, "Fear not, stand firm, and see the salvation of the LORD, which he will work for you today. For the Egyptians whom you see today, you shall never see again. The LORD will fight for you, and you have only to be silent."
>
> Exodus 14:13–14

Healthy Habit Helpers

1. Name the major battles going on in your life right now:

_____

_____

_____

2. After we pray, record any strategies God gives you for each battle (e.g., war, withdraw, wait, etc.):

_____

_____

_____

Now put your hand on your heart and pray this aloud with me:

Dear God, I resign as the general on the battlefields of my life and declare that You are in control of each battle. I surrender to You my demand for justice and declare my trust in You for vindication and protection. I trust You with my relationships, my community, my involvements and my nation. In Jesus' name I pray, Amen.

9

Keep Good Company

Show me your friends and I'll show you your future.

You have heard that phrase so many times it has lost its capacity to convict you. So let me say it like this: "Show me your three closest friends and I'll show you yourself in three years."

Are you hanging out with people who change their worlds through prayer? Then you will become a world-changing intercessor, too. Are you hanging out with people who complain and find coping mechanisms to muddle through? Then you will wind up a coping mechanism–muddler, too.

Who are your three closest friends? These are not people you met last week. These are friends who know all your secrets and who have seen you at your best and your worst. You spend a great deal of time with them, whenever able (in person, on the phone, online or all of them).

Now let me ask you three questions about your top three friends. Take this test for each of them individually. You are going to answer each question with (1) no, never, (2) 30 percent of the time, (3) 60 percent of the time or (4) 100 percent of the time.

a. Is he or she vocal about loving Jesus Christ with all the mind, soul, heart and strength? (Luke 10:27)

b. Does he or she seek first the Kingdom of God and all its righteousness? (Matthew 6:33—in other words, does he or she prioritize God and a right relationship with Him above every other activity or relationship?)

c. Is he or she planted in a local church, attending faithfully and flourishing there? (Psalm 92:13)

Now give your friend one point for each (1) they got, two points for each (2) and so on for all three questions. (In other words, if you answered "no, never," then give your friend one point on that question. If you answered "100 percent of the time," then score four.) The highest score for this test is 12 and the lowest is 3.

If your closest friend(s) scored 3–6 on this test, you can fully expect that in just a little while, you will no longer be vocal about loving Jesus with all your mind, soul, heart and strength, will not be seeking first the Kingdom and all its righteousness (you will not be in "right standing" with God) nor will you be planted *firmly* at the church God has called you to.

In short, this person does not need to be one of your closest friends.

If one of your friends scored 7–9, that is definitely better than 3 or 6, but you still might end up loving Jesus Christ with half of your heart, half of your mind and half of your strength, or seeking second (or third) the Kingdom of God, or missing more church than you attend.

If you have a friend on your close friends list who scores 9–12, God has sent you a most precious gift. Nourish that friendship. If you had such a friend at one time and walked away from that relationship and toward another more compromising one, then you rejected a gift from God. Tell Him you are sorry. Rekindle that relationship. *Today.* Tell that person he or she scored high on the *Healthy Living Handbook* friends test and that you need that person in your life. Fill your life with 12s! If you can only find one 12, you have found a lot. And four 3s are not the same as one 12. God's standard and His math do not work like that. There is no room on your close friends list for a 3. You will wind up taking his or her counsel, which is less than God's best. Listen to the very first Psalm:

> Blessed is the man that walketh not in the counsel of the ungodly, nor standeth in the way of sinners, nor sitteth in the seat of the scornful. But his delight is in the law of the LORD; and in his law doth he meditate day and night. And he shall be like a tree planted by the rivers of water, that bringeth forth his fruit in his season; his leaf also shall not wither; and whatsoever he doeth shall prosper. The ungodly are not so: but are like the chaff which the wind driveth away. Therefore the ungodly shall not stand in the judgment, nor sinners in the congregation of the righteous. For the LORD knoweth the way of the righteous: but the way of the ungodly shall perish.
>
> Psalm 1:1–6 KJV

Simply put, if we walk, stand or sit with people whose sole focus is something other than God, we will soon suffer that same fate because we are taking these friends' counsel, one life issue at a time. If you were raised a 12 or became one (pursuing God with your whole heart) and then decide to surround yourself with 3s as close friends, you may think you are pulling them up, but the truth is they are pulling you down. These are not just peripheral relationships. These are your closest counselors and advice givers! Before long no one can see the 12 you once were because now your friendships have averaged you down to a 5. Psalm 1 mentions avoiding the ungodly, the sinner and the scornful. It says we will be more blessed if we do. Theirs is a

165

life of judgment and perishing, and ours is a life of fruitfulness and prosperity. What is the opposite of the ungodly, sinners and the scornful? The godly, righteous and respectful. Those are the 12s you should surround yourself with, in your friendships and in selecting a spouse, as well.

So what *do* you do with these longtime friends who you know are not God's best for your life? You move them off the three closest friends list and onto a general friends list. They no longer get weekly or even monthly time with you, online, on the phone or in person. If you are aiming to influence this person for Christ, then you must first get to a stronger place in your faith again. I hate to keep using numeric equations, but they are concrete: If you were once a 12 and started hanging out with a top three of all 3s, it brought you down to a 5. So, before you do anything else, you need a lineup of 12s in your life to get you back where you were. *Then* you can add your 12 to others and raise them upward to the real, undiluted Gospel.

> **What is the opposite of the ungodly, sinners and the scornful? The godly, righteous and respectful.**

If God's Word is not enough to convince you that you should not be walking, standing, sitting or taking counsel from anyone other than godly, righteous, respectable people of faith, I want to also give you a list of warning signs for your relationships. Let's call this the "seven warning signs of a spiritually dangerous friendship." You know you are in a spiritually dangerous relationship if the friend in question:

1. Tends to be isolated and dependent on you, meaning you literally may be the only good friend he has and he is fine with that.
2. Tells you what you want to hear.

3. Believes in you so strongly that she would allow you to rebel against authority and say nothing to you.

4. Does not consistently compel you to walk a deeper walk with Jesus Christ and never mentions God's Word to you.

5. Tends to easily fall out of Christian fellowship, church, etc.

6. Is not a Christian, and you are trying to be.

7. Is often pessimistic or negative (as opposed to full of faith).

You know who these people are in your life. Be brave enough to turn them over to God while you regain your spiritual footing. Have the courage to say, "Good-bye for now." If they think so highly of you, they very well may follow you right to the foot of the cross. Stock your life with "shelves of 12s"!

I pray all the time for my children's relationships. I have prayed for many a friend of theirs and weighed each on the scales opposite my child to discern if they were equally yoked in their spiritual fervor. Better yet is for the friend to be even weightier in the Spirit than my child, so that his or her grounding influence would result in my child going even higher on the scales. If this friend is not as "weighty" in faith, then my child will surely sink in his or hers. Yes, I want my kids to influence the faithless, but I do not want those faithless ones included in their circle of counselors.

I have seen the enemy repeatedly try to plant friends with weightless faiths into my children's lives with the intention of sinking them. It is in my nature to trust my child, young or old (and, thus, the new friend), but if the Lord alerts me to a dangerous match, I immediately begin praying three things: (1) I ask God to give my child a discerning spirit to see the danger without my help. (2) If that does not work, then I pray for my child to lose favor with this individual so that the relationship ends. (3) If neither of those work—and this is always a last resort—then I pray for God to move this friend far, far away, leaving room for the "iron sharpening iron" friend that God wants in his or her place. I then begin calling that new friend forth as if it were a child of my own. I do this out loud and often with fasting. I have seen it work over and over and over in my maternal ministry to my children. Ungodly friends are choking weeds in a Christian mother's well-tended garden.

I obviously got the 30-60-100 scoring for the friends test from the Mark 4 passage of the Parable of the Sower, which we discussed in Healthy Living Habit No. 6 for your spirit, "Put On Your Sunday Shoes." I encourage you to go back and read it again when you are done here. I leave you with these Scriptures:

Don't be fooled: "Bad friends will ruin good habits." Come back to your right way of thinking and stop sinning.

1 Corinthians 15:33–34 EASY

Whoever walks with the wise becomes wise, but the companion of fools will suffer harm.

Proverbs 13:20

Do not be unequally yoked with unbelievers. For what partnership has righteousness with lawlessness? Or what fellowship has light with darkness?

2 Corinthians 6:14

I meant that you are not to associate with anyone who claims to be a believer yet indulges in sexual sin, or is greedy, or worships idols, or is abusive, or is a drunkard, or cheats people. Don't even eat with such people.

1 Corinthians 5:11 NLT

Healthy Habit Helpers

1. Name your three closest friends. Name those who need to move off that list and who should replace them:

_____

_____

_____

Now put your hand on your heart and pray this aloud with me:

God, first of all, You are my best friend. Forgive me for any substitutions I have made for You, and tell me who is not Your best for me. Show me who are to be my closest friends, those who will both comfort and confront me. In Jesus' name, Amen.

10

Bury the Hatchet

Do you know what these people have in common? Socrates, Cleopatra, Pope Clement II and Adolf Hitler: They and many other household names died after ingesting poison. The poisons used varied from cyanide to hemlock to asp venom.

Unforgiveness, like poison, comes in multiple varieties, but all are deadly to the soul. *Resentment is like drinking poison and waiting for the other person to die.* That phrase has been used so often it is almost impossible to trace its origin, but early on it was attributed to Malachy Gerard McCourt, an Irish-American Bible salesman turned actor, writer and politician. The implication is that we do not comprehend the poison we ingest each time we choose resentment over forgiveness.

Evidently, such unforgiveness is not only deadly to the soul, but to the body. In a 2012 article in CBN News' *Health and Science* column, Dr. Steven Standiford, chief of surgery at the Cancer Treatment Centers of America (CTCA), explained why the CTCA takes emotional health so seriously that it offers forgiveness therapy to treat cancer and other diseases: "It's important to treat emotional wounds or disorders because they really can hinder someone's reactions to the treatments, even someone's willingness to pursue treatment."[1] Refusing to forgive keeps people sick; evidently, of all cancer patients, a shocking 61 percent have forgiveness issues, and of those, more than half are extreme. That is according to Dr. Michael Barry, a pastor and author of *The Forgiveness Project*. He says that most who are under a heavy burden of hatred, unforgiveness and anger do not even realize it until they release it and forgive.[2]

Johns Hopkins University agrees. Karen Swartz, M.D., director of the Mood Disorders Adult Consultation Clinic at the Johns Hopkins Hospital, says, "There is an enormous physical burden to being hurt and disappointed."[3] You know this to be true in your own life. You have a fight with your spouse or parents or maybe just your neighbor. Suddenly, you are nauseous and sighing deeply, and your head hurts. Or maybe you are wronged financially or your reputation is maligned and the injustice is almost more than you can emotionally bear. Whenever the bitter memory comes to mind, you can feel the anger simmering in the pit of your stomach, or perhaps you carry the emotional tension in your back. You are experiencing the burden of disappointment. Dr. Swartz elaborates that repeated anger puts you into fight-or-flight mode, which results in physiological changes in heart rate, blood pressure and even your immune responses. Each of those leaves you quite vulnerable to a myriad of illnesses, including heart disease, diabetes and depression. Forgiveness appears to provide a barrier of protection to your health.

1. Lorie Johnson, "Holding Grudges? Forgiveness Key to Healthy Body," *CBN News Health and Science*, January 1, 2012, http://www.cbn.com/cbnnews/health science/2011/june/holding-grudges-forgiveness-key-to-healthy-body/?mobile=fa lse.

2. Ibid.

3. "Forgiveness: Your Health Depends on It," Johns Hopkins Medicine, http:// www.hopkinsmedicine.org/health/healthy_aging/healthy_connections/forgive ness-your-health-depends-on-it.

Bury the hatchet means to settle a difference with an adversary. The practice predates the European settlement of America, among Native American tribes who laid down their weapons (hatchets) as an act of peace. The New England Historical and Genealogical Register for 1870 has a record made by Samuel Sewall in 1680 in which he recounts the burying of hatchets by the indigenous peoples:

> Meeting wth ye Sachem [the tribal leaders] the[y] came to an agreemt and buried two Axes in ye Ground; which ceremony to them is more significant & binding than all Articles of Peace the Hatchet being a principal weapon wth ym.[4]

Although the phrase is never mentioned in Scripture, there are plenty of hatchet-buriers in the Bible. How difficult it must have been for Joseph to forgive his brothers, who had thrown him into the pit and sold him into slavery. After the pit and servitude in Potiphar's house came the false accusations that led to his imprisonment. At all of those junctures, Joseph had ample time to sit and think, *I would not be here if not for those traitors!* Or, *Why did You forget me, O God?* Surely he plotted his revenge, or at least his vindication. I probably would have. But that is not what readily flowed from Joseph's heart when his brothers came to him in need. Food was scarce in a region-wide famine, and they had traveled for provision all the way to Egypt, where Joseph had been elevated to second

Whenever the bitter memory comes to mind, you can feel the anger simmering in the pit of your stomach, or perhaps you carry the emotional tension in your back. You are experiencing the burden of disappointment.

4. "The Meaning and Origin of the Expression: Bury the Hatchet," The Phrase Finder, accessed May 25, 2017, http://www.phrases.org.uk/meanings/bury-the-hatchet.html.

in command behind Pharaoh after just one solid dream interpretation. They did not recognize Joseph, but he knew them. Through Joseph's forgiveness and mercy, God saved a people. He saved Egypt. He saved Israel. He saved you! You see, Genesis 37:26 tells us that it was his brother Judah who had the idea to sell Joseph into slavery. Yet when Judah stood before him with his hand out for food, Joseph, who could have easily had him killed, forgave. Had he not, the Lion of the tribe of *Judah*—our Messiah, Jesus—might never have been born. The moral of this story is that God had not forsaken Joseph at all; in fact, it appeared **Unforgiveness could** that it was God Himself who orchestrated **have prevented Jesus'** everything, taking him from the bosom of **prophesied birth.** his family to preserve it. But the divine plan would have collapsed without forgiveness. Unforgiveness could have prevented Jesus' prophesied birth.

I desire to learn the art of such lavish and lenient forgiveness. My heart often requires more of a running start, predictably finding its way there after much deliberation and soul searching, and I wonder if it will ever be as effortless as I desire it to be. But what I do not want is to arrive in heaven one day only to face a conversation with Joseph in which he explains to me something that my unforgiveness cost me, or my children, or my grandchildren. Maybe there are no tears in heaven, but there is truth, and I want my truth to include that I loved forgiveness and mercy more than the temporary pleasure that justice brings my flesh.

Many years ago I had an opportunity to take part in a special meeting celebrating the coming together of the Tennessee government and spiritual leaders to create an official resolution that would ask forgiveness for the atrocities committed against the Native Americans through the Trail of Tears, initiated at the pen of President Andrew Jackson. But the morning of the meeting I was blindsided by sickness and in bed most of the day. I believed it was spiritual warfare to keep me from going, but when I sought the Lord, He told me it was not. I asked God why this had passed through His hand to me, and I was hit with the sobering thought that it would be dangerous—if not impossible—to stand before a Holy God that evening to corporately ask His forgiveness for the egregious sins of previous Tennesseans if I was harboring unforgiveness in my own heart toward anyone. I could not fool God, or the enemy. If unforgiveness is a demonic force—which I believe it is—how could I entertain it in my heart and yet cast it out of someone else's? The enemy would know. I knew I needed to come clean before the meeting, and so I decided to make a forgiveness list. That breezy spring afternoon I sat in my backyard by my flower garden, asking God to bring to mind anyone in my heart that I had not forgiven over the years. I honestly did not think there was anything of significance. But as I began to relive my life—starting at a very young age—I began to feel the "burden of disappointment." The tears came. Even though by this point I had only lived about four and a half decades on this earth, I had spent half of it in ministry, and with that comes frequent rejection and disappointment. People love you when they are making vows for growth and feeling God's presence, but when they break those vows, they begin rejecting everyone who heard them made, which usually includes their pastors. With these stories, departures and rejections filling up the front and back side of my paper, the list was soon more than two hundred people. I had *not* been walking around with anxious, vengeful thoughts about any of them, but I was shocked at how much hurt my heart had endured. It felt so good to let it all go. I felt joy come from this obedience, and God's pleasure followed. So did the perfect health that allowed me to attend the meeting that night. After making my list, I took the pages and burned them, and, as if by providence, the breeze carried the ashes into my garden. I took the remaining ones and scattered them onto a small bush my father had given me but that had never flowered, and, sure enough, that summer it bloomed so full that the colorful flowers overpowered almost every trace of green.

Now that I have given you some examples of what forgiveness is, let me tell you some things it is not. (I have set these to the acronym *FORGIVE*.) Forgiveness is not:

Forgetting. To forgive is not to forget. But forgetting can miraculously happen!

Overlooking. You are not denying the hurt. You name it, but forgive it.

Reducing. You are not minimizing the offense by forgiving it.

Gossiping. You cannot truly forgive and keep speaking ill of the offender.

Ignoring. You are giving your full attention to this hurt and forgiving it.

Vindicating. You are not trying to vindicate yourself. But vindication may come another way.

Excusing. You are not making excuses for the offender, but forgiving him or her.

Forgiveness is a spiritual force that is anything but weak or accidental. It is deliberate and strong. It is like a giant pair of scissors that cuts you loose from death—body, mind and spirit. Emotionally healthy people forgive.

Consider this Scripture, and study the passages that follow it: "Be kind to one another, tenderhearted, forgiving one another, as God in Christ forgave you" (Ephesians 4:32). Other passages to study: Romans 12:14; Mark 11:25; Matthew 6:15; 1 John 1:9; Matthew 18:21–22; Matthew 6:14–15; Luke 6:27; Colossians 3:13.

Healthy Habit Helpers

1. Make your own forgiveness list on a separate sheet. Afterward, burn the list and scatter the ashes (outside or in your fireplace). Then put your hand on your heart and pray this with me:

God, first forgive me for my unforgiveness. I forgive these people with all my heart. I acknowledge the tears, hurt and anger, but I release it all right now in Jesus' name. I forgive. I fully pardon them. Now fill my heart with new thoughts about them, Lord. Help me. Help them. Help us. Amen.

Section 3

The Top 10 Healthy Living Habits for Your *Body*

1

"Let Food Be Thy Medicine"

Hippocrates—father of the Hippocratic oath, which serves as an ethical medical standard for all physicians—said, "Let food be thy medicine." I am not antimedicine by any means; my life has been saved because of it. But I know no physician who would disagree with Hippocrates' incredible fifth- and sixth-century findings of the power in prescribing diet, exercise, massage and more to help treat disease.

An upcoming healthy living habit is entitled "Eat the Rainbow." What do you think of when you hear that title? I hope not Skittles or M&M's! That title refers to filling your plate each meal with all the beautiful colors God has put into our fruits and vegetables. Did you know that He made those colors for your health? Did you know you cannot be healthy if you do not consume them? Are you aware that each fruit or vegetable's color is a divinely intentional invention and does not merely represent the creative mood God was in at the moment He created it? That color is a miraculous result of specific phytonutrients and their pigments. They are put there to protect the plant from disease and harmful environmental toxins and to give it longevity of life, so just imagine what happens when you eat it! Most amazingly, each color specifically ministers to and cleanses specific organs. God has color-coded your foods.

Although I am a farmer's daughter and a farmer's granddaughter (both my maternal and paternal grandparents ran farms for a living, and my parents both grew up working on them), I admit that I had no idea about the color-cure connection until I wrote *The 30-Day Faith Detox: Renew Your Mind, Cleanse Your Body, Heal Your Spirit* in 2014. Or, I should say, I had no idea why certain foods are the color they are until I almost lost my life in 2012, after discovering I was on the brink of adrenal failure and had to use food for medicine. You have reached stage 4 of adrenal fatigue (a.k.a. adrenal exhaustion, adrenal burnout, Addison's disease) when all of your organs completely shut down due to the depletion of the important hormones adrenaline and cortisol. By the time I was diagnosed, I was already in stage 3. In my case, I had blown out my adrenal glands through the lack of deep, restorative, healing sleep, and most of my organs had begun to shut down, confirmed by multiple blood, urine and saliva tests. Because my liver was one of the organs in such bad shape, and because the liver is responsible for helping break down substances that we take by mouth, I could not just begin taking umpteen prescription drugs to bolster each organ, or else my liver might very well have gone on full-blown strike. Instead, I had to eat strategically in order to live. I did take certain natural dietary supplements, but they were layered in as my body could handle them and overseen by a master nutritionist.

God has color-coded your foods.

It was during this time that I "accidentally" (providentially) began to notice certain color patterns as I was working to heal each organ. Reds are good for the heart. Purples are good for treating pulmonary issues and the lungs. Why had

180

no one ever told me these things? Wait, did the majority of the world even know? Did my grandparents know? Did doctors know? God knew. I suddenly wanted to tell everyone. Creating each lifesaving meal became like studying and taking a final exam, three times a day. Being on full bed rest made that research easier, but standing and cooking it was out of the question, so I passed along the information to the people at my church, who were preparing meals for us, and suddenly the entire church was having to learn to "cook the rainbow." As a result, a health revolution started at our church. While some had already been health conscious, others were definitely not, and suddenly—with the sole motivation of helping their pastor/friend live—we were all on the same nutritional page. Eastgate Creative Christian Fellowship turned into a lean, mean nutrition machine. Not everyone, of course, but the atmosphere became supercharged with culinary chatter and recipe revelations. We were like-minded believers on a mission to live long and live strong, and this newfound mission even found its way into our children's department, where we rid our menu of all sugar and wheat boxed snacks and replaced them with a healthy, organic, all-fruit menu. It was not in the budget, but we put it there by faith. Sure enough, it and the other changes we made attracted new families, and our church grew, which more than covered the costs of that faith investment.

As a final cherry on top, *The 30-Day Faith Detox* was birthed out of this revolution, and my pastoring took on a whole new dimension, that being that I now felt responsible before God for my flock's diet. Imagine that. Should not every good shepherd care what his sheep eat? I suddenly did. I also began to feel the weight of this burden for the entire Body of Christ, and given that I was an author with a book-publishing contract, I just knew that Jehovah Sneaky was going to require me to write about it all. Feeling that I owed it to my readers to give them more than just personal experience, I decided to go back to school after my full recovery (which was in record time, by the way), and I became a certified nutritional counselor. It was also the impetus behind continuing on toward my degree in original medicine.

It was at this point that I learned the nutritional secrets that I am going to pass along to you in this section. The earth's thousands of species of fruits and vegetables all contain various phytonutrients that, when combined, constitute the perfect prevention for any ailment that might try to afflict you and the perfect aid for whatever already has.

Eastgate Creative Christian Fellowship turned into a lean, mean nutrition machine.

Think of it: God created man, and where did He put him? In a garden. And what was God's original diet? Listen to Genesis 1:29 (KJV): "And God said, Behold, I have given you every herb bearing seed, which is upon the face of all the earth, and every tree, in the which is the fruit of a tree yielding seed; to you it shall be for meat."

Very interesting! For one thing, He reveals here that He is giving them (and us) every plant and fruit from the trees for food—but He also refers to that food as "meat." Does that mean that God intends us to eat only vegetables and not animal flesh for meat? We will explore this "vegetarian theology" (my witticism) in an upcoming healthy living habit and see how it holds up scripturally and nutritionally; but for now I want us to concentrate on the miracle of plant-based foods and how we should utilize them as "medicine." From Scripture we see an indisputable fact: God created our most nutritional foods on the third day of creation. And, curiously, there is also something we *do not* see in Scripture: cooking in the Garden of Eden.

Are you ready in this section to rethink the way you eat, sleep, breathe and move? Well, then, enjoy this poem, answer the quick questions, pray the prayer and let's get started!

Good Nutrition

I'd like to give you food for thought if you'll give me
  permission
And possibly it could offend (I have a keen suspicion)
But these few words might wake you up and set you on a
  mission
Since helping you live long and strong is purely my ambition
It's time you take back your physique and give it definition
Stop pigging out, start working out and lose your inhibition
Start walking, running, stepping and do body demolition
Stop acting like those long-lost curves are just an apparition

Get serious about your chow and call a dietician
Or someone who can take your fork and give an admonition
Then count your carbs and calories as if you're a tactician
And chew your food well as you eat and take an
  intermission!
Take vitamins and supplements and contact your physician
Especially if underweight and suffering malnutrition
Start viewing food as medicine and snacks as ammunition
Take back your bod and whip it into absolute submission

It's possible to get a plan and make a smart transition
It starts with just awareness and an honest, frank admission
Then tell your friends and family and make some new
  traditions
Then watch your whole anatomy receive a recondition
The time is now for you to give your Maker recognition
He crafted you one of a kind, a limited edition
So start today with hope and claim your sunny disposition
It's waiting for you on the other side of good nutrition.
©Laura Harris Smith

Healthy Habit Helpers

1. Do you have any illnesses you are currently fighting? If so, what?

_____

_____

_____

_____

2. Exactly how are you fighting them? (Not fighting the symptoms only, but the disease itself to work toward its elimination.)

_____

_____

_____

_____

Now put your hand over your heart and pray this aloud with me:

Father God, thank You for my body. Even with all of its struggles—past and present—it has seen me through these decades of life and I am thankful for it. Help me help it house Your Holy Spirit, Lord! My body is Your temple! Thank You for every modern medical treatment and medication that may have seen me thus far, but, Father, teach me here and now how to walk in divine health so that I am not always in need of healing. My spirit is willing but my flesh is weak, so guide me through this section and make me a physically healthy person. I pray this all in Your name, Jesus, Amen.

2

Eat the Rainbow

I have never found that bush I am supposed to beat around, so let me get right to the point: You know you are supposed to eat your vegetables. You think about it. You hear the statistics and stories of what happens to people who omit them—and fruits— from their diets. Their hearts fail sooner and they succumb to cardiovascular disease death. Their blood sugar goes wonky faster, resulting in diabetes and obesity. The lack of cruciferous fiber means their digestive tracts are never cleansed, putting them at risk for colon cancer. Their cholesterol rises and their immune system function plummets, leaving them wide open to all sorts of infirmity. Their skin ages quicker, making them look forty at thirty, fifty at forty and so on. So, if you know all these things, then *why are you still in vegetable rebellion?*

If I were to say, "Use this shampoo and you will have forty-two percent fewer bad hair days and never die from embarrassment from a bad photo again!" you would do it. But if I say, "Eat your daily fruits and veggies and lower your risk of dying from *anything* by forty-two percent," you might change the subject. It is the most bizarre phenomenon I have ever seen. People would rather have better hair days than length of days period. Because their insides are hidden, they do not realize the level of degeneration that is happening due to poor nutrition, and so they ignore it (until chronic sickness sets in and they get the wakeup call). But I believe in people. I believe that eventually those who truly love living will do what is necessary to keep living longer. Or let me be more blunt: I believe that eventually people who do not want to die will quit killing themselves. They will raise their forks as weapons and take back their health, one meal at a time.

"People who eat seven or more portions of vegetables and fruit a day have a 42 percent lower risk of dying from any cause, compared to those who eat less than one portion." ~Dr. Joseph Mercola

And the 42 percent figure is true; the research was published in the *Journal of Epidemiology and Community Health*. In a fascinating article entitled "Eating More Fruits and Vegetables Can Cut Your Risk of Dying in Half," Dr. Joseph Mercola discusses the findings of this study:

> People who eat seven or more portions of vegetables and fruit a day have a 42 percent lower risk of dying from any cause, compared to those who eat less than one portion. They also enjoy a 31 percent lower risk of heart disease and a 25 percent lower risk of cancer.[1]

In a 2016 article entitled, "Want to Die Sooner? Then Don't Eat Your Vegetables," research on the link between vegetable and fruit consumption and decreased mortality was outlined better than I have seen anywhere before.[2] It references a 2014 team of

1. Joseph Mercola, D.O., "Eating More Fruits and Vegetables Can Cut Your Risk of Dying in Half," Mercola.com, April 14, 2014, http://articles.mercola.com/sites/articles/archive/2014/04/14/eating-fruits-vegetables.aspx.
2. "Want to Die Sooner? Then Don't Eat Your Vegetables," PricePlow.com, June 28, 2016, https://blog.priceplow.com/vegetables.

Chinese and American researchers who conducted a "monstrous meta-analysis of diet and mortality data" that was published in *BMJ* (formerly known as the *British Medical Journal*). Here was the objective: "To examine and quantify the potential dose-response relation between fruit and vegetable consumption and risk of all cause, cardiovascular, and cancer mortality."[3] (My translation: Is "give me vegetables or give me death" true?)

The researchers carefully selected sixteen studies published in major medical journals from 1950 to 2013; each study ranged in duration from 4.6 to 26 years. The meta-analysis included an impressive 833,234 participants (all human, meaning animal studies were excluded). After finding potential studies that helped them with their objective, the researchers isolated the ones that dealt with various causes of death and then paired those with studies on fruit and vegetable intake. Again, the objective was to see what difference vegetable and fruit consumption really made to the length of people's lives in these studies. "Who ate what and died when?" so to speak. The results were amazing! The indisputable conclusion was that, yes, a diet high in fruits and vegetables leads to a longer life. In the researchers' words:

> Conclusions: This meta-analysis provides further evidence that higher consumption of fruit and vegetables is associated with a lower risk of mortality from all causes, particularly from cardiovascular diseases. The results support current recommendations to increase consumption to promote health and overall longevity.[4]

The study also found that for each additional serving of vegetables or fruit, the risk of dying from cardiovascular disease

3. Xia Wang, Yingying Ouyand, Jun Liu, Minmin Zhu, Gang Zhao, Wei Bao, and Frank B. Hu, *BMJ* 349 (2014), http://www.bmj.com/content/bmj/349/bmj.g4490.full.pdf.
4. Ibid.

drops by 5 percent. But you cannot just keep racking up the 5 percent bonus chips and live forever. It seems the benefits cap out at a threshold of five total servings a day, at which point the risk of heart disease–related death is lowered by 26 percent. But what good news! God has put the power in our hands to live long and strong, one meal at a time!

Interestingly, fruits "outperformed" vegetables, showing that each additional serving of fruit decreased the likelihood of heart disease death by 6 percent versus 5 percent for veggies. So no skimping on fruits.

But how many fruits and vegetables should you eat daily? Well, in all of my nutritional schooling and in the research and texts I have studied in recent years, I have learned that most nutritional experts agree that the diet should be composed of 75 percent vegetables and fruits. If they do not agree with that, they certainly never say 75 percent is bad for you! Experts differ on what portion of your 75 percent should be cooked or eaten raw, but the number remains consistent. It is not at all the RDA—recommended daily allowance—food pyramid we were raised on. It is instead the "ODA," or "optimum daily allowance."

People tend to get lost in the "how many servings per day?" rule. If you will just aim to eat 2–3 cups of fruit a day and 2–3 cups of vegetables a day *at minimum*, you are off to a good start. Or just think of that 75 percent goal for each plate you are preparing for yourself. Fill up each plate or bowl with 75 percent cooked and/or fresh vegetables. The other arguments over meat and wheat contributing the other 25 percent pale in comparison when this healthy 75 percent veggie and fruit rule is kept.

But what if you hate vegetables or fruits or just do not like many of them? You are going to love the next healthy living habit, "Watch Your Mouth," because your solution awaits.

If you find it difficult to get in your ODA of vegetables and fruits each day, then how about daily smoothies? They are versatile, creative, healthy and require no cooking! I even offer a Custom Smoothie service on LauraHarrisSmith.com so that you can have a tailor-made smoothie recipe created by me for your unique physical needs. We will talk more about that in our next healthy living habit, too.

The amazing thing about our creative God is that He has color-coded our fruits and vegetables so that we can know for sure that we are giving our bodies exactly what they need. Red fruits and vegetables are red not just because God was in a bold mood at the moment He created them but because they contain a phytonutrient called lycopene. Red lycopene is especially good for the heart (easy to remember, right?). It is good for other organs as well, but it is generally advertised as a heart-healthy supplement, and rightfully so. But it is so much easier, healthier, cheaper and tastier just to reach for red grapes or red peppers or a strawberry! Plus, the fruits and vegetables will act like claws and detoxify your body, whereas one pill will not.

> I even offer a Custom Smoothie service on LauraHarrisSmith.com so that you can have a tailor-made smoothie recipe created by me for your unique physical needs.

For a full education about which organs are cleansed and detoxified by which color foods (and why), I urge you to do the total body detox offered in my last book, *The 30-Day Faith Detox: Renew Your Mind, Cleanse Your Body, Heal Your Spirit.* All fifteen of your major body systems will be cleansed by the end of the thirty days. Along with its thirty spiritual devotionals and prayers for emotional healing from faith toxins, you will have experienced a total temple cleansing. Imagine a reset button for your body, mind and spirit, and join the tens of thousands of individuals all over the world who are doing the faith detox and losing weight, gaining faith and improving the quality of their lives.

Healthy Habit Helpers

1. Roughly what percentage of your diet is plant based? (Goal is 75 percent for a healthy, long life.) And what is your favorite vegetable and favorite fruit?

_____

_____

_____

_____

_____

Now put your hand over your heart and pray this aloud with me:

God, I ask You to help me make the dietary changes I need to live a long life. Forgive me for expecting You to override my poor food choices and for abusing my body, which is Your temple. Change starts today. Amen!

3

Watch Your Mouth

Anybody else but me hear that phrase growing up? Well, speech is important, but the truth is that we should watch our mouths for much more than just making sure that our conversations are always filled with honor. We should also govern every bite that goes into them as if our lives depends on it. Because they do.

Bad dietary habits are more easily hidden in your teens and twenties because of "reserves," but as the nutrient-depleted body matures, it ages (dies) faster than it should, just like a flower or leaf cut from its vine of nourishment does not show visible signs of shriveling at first but then withers exponentially as the days go on. So the young person mentally develops decades' worth of self-deceiving belief in invincibility, only to find strange health changes occurring around his or her thirties. The aging process advances very quickly at this point because, as of the thirties, the hormone peak has passed and is now on the decline. There is no cosmetic for this type of aging, and there is certainly no cosmetic for the aging taking place on the inside. It is a disturbing phase because people are not doing anything differently than they have for decades, and yet now something seems wrong. Something was always wrong, but now the body is demanding attention. And payment.

In this healthy living habit we are going to briefly discuss the top three foods I get asked about as a nutritionist, which are "meat, wheat and sweets." Then we will see how you can fashion your speech so that what comes out of your mouth will actually assist you in making better choices about what goes in it. "Watch your mouth!"

> **Meat.** Much can be said about meat consumption—and I will say more in the next healthy living habit, when we will be discussing processed and fast foods (which contain mainly meat). In a nutshell, though, many believe that Scripture points to God's original design for diet not including meat, and that it was only added for a short period right after the Flood, when all plant vegetation had died. What food did Noah have right on the ark? Meat. That theory, coupled with the fact that vegetarians live longer than meat eaters, is a compelling argument for what some consider to be a vegetarian theology.

> **Wheat.** Gluten, a mixture of two proteins found in wheat (and certain other grains), is the "glue" that makes bread doughy. Today's wheat is not the wheat from six thousand, six hundred or even sixty years ago. For lower costs and greater profit, modern grain processors learned to separate the nutritious components of grain (the bran and germ) from the endosperm, where most of the carbohydrates are. This modification resulted in a sharp reduction in nutrition content, not to mention that today's refined bread can contain up to ten times more gluten than yesteryear's bread did, something our bodies were never designed by God to digest. So they do not, meaning that many times the gluten just sits in your gut and rots. All the "refining"

also results in sharp blood sugar spikes that put strain on the rest of the body. There are nineteen other grains/flours out there besides wheat, so my advice is to experiment and find the ones you like! My favorites are almond flour and brown rice flour, and I have not missed wheat a bit in these last five years because of all the options. I do not have celiac disease, but I do feel much better off of wheat, and I guarantee you will, too! And bye-bye wheat belly!

Sweets. Oh, how I wish that the stevia plant had been discovered before the sugarcane. The world would have less diabetes and obesity. Refined sugars are bad for numerous reasons. They not only lead to diabetes and obesity, but also higher cholesterol, liver overload, insulin resistance and even cancer. Oh, and let's not forget that sugar is highly addictive. Please (pretty please) let this be the season that you experiment with healthy sweeteners like stevia, xylitol and agave. If you use honey, use it very rarely and in minimal amounts. Experiment with various forms of stevia until you find the right one. It comes in powder, leaves and liquid, and it does not take much stevia to sweeten a food because the leaves are up to seventy times sweeter than sugar, while the powder is two to three hundred times sweeter. If you get too much, you will get a strong aftertaste and think you do not like stevia. You do! You may just not know it yet!

So what *do* you eat if you are eating little to no wheat, meat or sweets? Obviously, we are right back to eating the rainbow. You must aim to have 75 percent of your daily food intake be fruits and vegetables if you want to live long and live strong. If you want to live out all the days God has for you, then you have to eat the foods He has told you in Scripture that He has made for you: "And God said, 'Behold, I have given you every plant yielding seed that is on the face of all the earth, and every tree with seed in its fruit. You shall have them for food'" (Genesis 1:29).

Dread vegetables and fruits? Consider yourself a picky-tarian? I have a few ideas for you: First and foremost, quit saying you hate vegetables. Quit saying you hate any healthy food! And stop saying how much you love sugar and cannot live without wheat bread. The power of life and death is in your tongue, and every time you say these things you are reinforcing the problem. Do not reject the gift of God through the plants of the fields! God Himself is the one who has given these fruits and vegetables to you, and it was for good cause, for in them are the medicinal cures necessary for your total well-being.

Second, remember that there are hundreds of thousands of different vegetables and fruits out there for you to try. There are more than 7,500 different species of apples alone! So do not get discouraged. Search for new fruits and vegetables as if you are searching for gold, for that is what they are.

Third, for the next four weeks I want you to buy a new vegetable each week from the grocery. Bring it home and find a creative way to prepare it. (Default: smother it in olive oil and pink salt and roast it in your oven for 30 minutes at 375 degrees.) After that, do it all over again for another four weeks. Do it every week this year, and by the end of the year you will have tried 52 new vegetables or fruits (and herbs!), and because you have had total creative control over preparation, the chances are good that you *will like* some and keep buying them!

Fourth, hide your vegetables in other foods. Puree them in casseroles, grind them up in gravies and so on. And remember the "fork load method," which is taking a bite of vegetables or fruits along with something else on your plate that you do love.

Finally, pray my Veggie Hater's Prayer at the end of this commentary. Pray it over yourself daily if you must, but do it! I have heard of *amazing* results from people who told me that God entirely changed their palate with this prayer, when mixed with faith.

Tip: Try to get a good chunk of your fruits and vegetables in for the day at breakfast. That way, you do not have to worry about counting all day, and besides, you will have much more sustainable time-released energy if you do! We talked in "Eat the Rainbow" about smoothies. The reason I mention it again is twofold. First, you can hide a ton inside a smoothie (things you like and things you dislike), and it is relatively easy to make. You can assemble most of the ingredients the night before in a mason jar, then seal and place it in your refrigerator. It saves time for the next morning, and then you can pour the blended smoothie right back in the same mason jar to drink on the road or at home.

Second, I so believe in the power of smoothies that I want to help you create the perfect one for your own body's physical needs. Just go to LauraHarrisSmith.com/Custom_Smoothies .html, place "Custom Smoothie" in your cart, check out and then wait to receive your health questionnaire by email. You will list your health issues or needs, and I will then personalize a smoothie just for you that will target the areas that need healing help in your body. You will be emailed a colorful recipe with your name on it to show your friends and family—a smoothie named after *you*! And the coolest part is that you will have this "prescription" breakfast (or snack) recipe for about what it costs to buy four smoothies somewhere else, and you can make it for yourself at home whenever you like. Win-win!

Again and again people ask my opinion on eating this or that food. My answer is that no food is going to keep you out of heaven. Of course, it might get you there sooner, and that is entirely your choice!

Healthy Habit Helpers

1. Name your three greatest dietary weaknesses below, and then list possible solutions:

_____

_____

_____

_____

_____

Now put your hand over your heart and pray this aloud with me:

God, I see from Your Word that You gave me vegetables and fruits as food. I want what You want for me, and I will not allow those dots on my tongue—my taste buds—to rule my life or determine how long I live. Change my palate, Lord, and help me begin to eat vegetables and fruits. I will do it by faith, God. But help me enjoy it. I lay aside my prejudice about vegetables and fruits and ask You to help me make better choices for a longer life. Color my plate, Lord. Amen.

4

Don't Eat and Run!

"Two all-beef patties, special sauce, lettuce, cheese, pickles, onions on a sesame seed bun." If you know what product that jingle advertises, give yourself two points. If you know the tune and can sing it, give yourself three points. But if you have ever *eaten* a Big Mac, take off *five* points!

How fortuitous that when I was taking a college speech class at Belmont University in the late 1980s (as a young mother), I chose to do my persuasive speech on the dangers of fast food. I was studying religion and theatre, and yet even then the job of instructing others about health and nutrition must have been calling my name. I had decided to take a speech class taught by a young, inspiring, encouraging professor named Dr. Jimmy Davis. I began that speech with the Big Mac jingle to get the class's attention, and then I added, ". . . equals seventy-nine grams of cholesterol, one thousand seven grams of sodium, forty-four grams of carbs and thirty-three grams of fat."

It got a chuckle, and it "hooked" them. In those days, nobody was talking about fast-food nutrition (or the lack thereof), but these fast food–junkie undergrads genuinely seemed on the edges of their seats. I then passed around a plate of items bought from fast-food restaurants that I had allowed to decompose. Trouble was, they never decomposed—they had just petrified into hockey pucks due to all the preservatives. If they do in your gut what they did on that plate, I would dare say that there is still residue in my digestive tract from all the fast food I ate in the 1980s! I got an A on that speech, and I actually kept the written version Dr. Davis graded, because in the margin he wrote, "Laura, you really should consider a career in public speaking." I remember laughing when I read that. But it obviously rang true in my spirit because I have kept that paper these thirty years. Turns out Dr. Davis was right! Public speaking, media appearances, teaching and preaching are how I make my living today—from the springboard of my writing—and I guess I even put that skill to use during my years as a TV host on the Shop At Home Network. Perhaps I will send Dr. Davis a copy of this book and say, "Thanks!"

So here I am again, attempting another persuasive speech on the dangers of fast-food consumption. Actually, in this healthy living habit we are going to discuss the dangers of fast food *and* the dangers of eating food fast. No more eating on the run!

I wrote in my last book, *The 30-Day Faith Detox*, "Mark my words . . . Processed foods are the new smoking. One day we will look back and wonder why we ever consumed them."[1] It is wiser by far to eat cleanly and colorfully, the combination of which can be achieved by eating locally. The fast foods you eat are shipped from who knows where and contain who knows what in terms of grades of meat and pesticide-laden produce. Conversely, foods you purchase at your local farmers' market or grocer's organic section, or that you grow yourself,

---

1. Laura Harris Smith, *The 30-Day Faith Detox: Renew Your Mind, Cleanse Your Body, Heal Your Spirit* (Minneapolis: Chosen, 2016), 23.

are toxin-free and will provide you with optimum health. To have whole health, you must eat whole foods.

If you think about it, it says a lot about our society that we must have food fast. To undo our addiction to fast food, we must first undo our addiction to speed. And impatience. Hey, I am a speed freak. I hate wasting time. Remember that I have already confessed to you that I alphabetize my spice cabinet because I hate wasting time on even the smallest details of disorganization. But I have had to reprogram my food-preparation clock. At one time my kitchen had *three* microwaves because it allowed me to defrost and cook a meal in record time for my huge family.[2] Once I began to look at the preparation time of the food as being just as enjoyable as the meal itself—and to include the family in it—I got rid of my countertop microwaves altogether. I especially treasure the moments spent chopping up fruits and vegetables for smoothies with my kiddos and standing around the blender tossing and talking.

> **To have whole health, you must eat whole foods.**

I dare say that our bodies are confused by the foreign products of modern food technology that we introduce to our gastrointestinal systems. Our bodies know it is not food. Although I am encouraged to see some fast-food chains coming around and changing their menus to include more color, we have no guarantee that the color is clean. Even if it is, it is still "fast" food when it is eaten on the run. Whether you are consuming fast food or consuming your food fast, neither will help you achieve good health. Yes, you will get more work done (business, school, even ministry), but how long will you get to enjoy the fruit of everything you are working so hard to build if you are not alive when it is completed? Today's processed foods (not just

2. For an in-depth investigation of the dangers of microwave radiation that I did myself in my own kitchen, *please* see the "Prepare Your Appliances" section on page 45 of *The 30-Day Faith Detox*.

fast foods, but also processed junk foods that line our grocery shelves) are nutrient deficient and lacking in enzymes, and they will eventually lead to digestive issues. You may say you have no digestive issues, but because 70 percent of your immune system is in your gut, a poor diet means a poorly operating immune system. So if you get sick, it could all be traced to your diet's lack of ability to protect you from that illness. Hippocrates said, "All disease begins in the gut."

So what are you putting in your gut? Mostly meat? Mostly bread or other refined, processed foods? Remember that 75 percent of your diet should be composed of fruits and vegetables if you want to live long—that is, 75 percent of each plate you serve, and many more interpret Scripture to say 100 percent.

Dr. Don Colbert is a *New York Times* bestselling author of more than forty books and has ministered health and healing to millions through his writings, frequent television appearances and online interviews. Dr. Colbert believes that Americans eat far too much meat, as do I and most other health experts. He says in his book *Toxic Relief: Restore Health and Energy through Fasting and Detoxification*,

> I recommend that women eat only 2 to 3 ½ ounces of lean, free-range meat, preferably only once daily, or at the most twice daily. Men, limit meats to only 3 ½ to 6 ½ ounces of lean, free-range meat, only one or, at the most, two times a day.[3]

But the meat and dairy industries have done a good job at convincing us that our protein requirements are much higher than that. We only need look to the miracle recipe of mother's milk, however, to see how our need for protein decreases over time. Breast milk is about 2.37 percent protein for the first six months of nursing, but the protein content decreases sharply

3. Don Colbert, M.D., *Toxic Relief: Restore Health and Energy through Fasting and Detoxification*, 2nd ed. (Lake Mary, Fla.: Siloam, 2012), 43.

to 1.07 percent at the six-month mark. This clearly indicates nature's built-in response to our dietary needs as we grow. As adults, we are "done" growing. We actually need only between 10 and 25 grams of protein a day, yet the standard American diet contains between 100 and 200 grams a day. Fast food plays a huge part in that. The Big Mac we sang about earlier has 26 grams of protein, which is well past your daily need (unless you want to keep "growing" and expand your waistline). Such excess protein from too much meat can result in weight gain, kidney problems, seizures, high blood levels of uric acid, liver enzyme issues and other smaller but harmful inconveniences like bad moods, bad breath and bad body odor (especially with a diet of mostly red meat and processed foods). Also, heavy meat eaters excrete more acidic urine because protein is high in sulfur and meat has a high phosphorus content; together these lead to a very acidic urine, which can develop into bladder cancer. If the acid is merely absorbed back into the muscles, it results in rheumatism (now called rheumatoid arthritis).

God has set certain natural laws in motion that He seems to respect. Too much sun burns. Too much rain floods. Too much processed food kills.

It brings me no pleasure to be the bearer of such news, and I assure you I am not into fearmongering. Jesus can heal anyone, anytime. But I also know God has set certain natural laws in motion that He seems to respect. Too much sun burns. Too much rain floods. Too much processed food kills.

Not even bodybuilders need tons of meat. Take the Swedish bodybuilder, Andreas Cahling, who won Mr. Pro International. He was a true frugivore, meaning he ate only fruit.[4] He consumed it before, during and after his training, abstaining from

4. Dr. Jim Sharps, N.D., H.D., Dr.NSc., Ph.D., *Basic Principles of Total Health* (Smithfield, Va.: International Institute of Original Medicine, 2011), 12.

all meat, dairy, grains and even vegetables (he did eat cucumbers, tomatoes and squash, since those are all seed-bearing plants and classify botanically as fruit). I would not call that an ideal diet, but it at least dispels the belief that you cannot build muscle without excess meat and protein.

As for the speed at which we ingest our food, many of us stuff our mouths, chew a few times and swallow fast so that we can continue on with the table conversation. The digestive tract is an amazing highway extending from the mouth to the rectum, and digestion begins in the mouth with the digestive enzymes in saliva. Have you noticed how your mouth waters when you think of your favorite foods? That is God's way of preparing your digestive juices so that with proper chewing (thirty chews for each bite of food) your food will enter your stomach in a more liquefied form, lessening the chance of reflux, gastroesophageal reflux disease, constipation and a myriad of other digestive issues. In your home you smell food cooking for an hour (or more), and your digestive juices are working overtime preparing to digest your food, whereas if you drive through a fast-food restaurant, you only get the first whiff when they open the window for payment. Always leave ample time to anticipate your food. Even praying over your food while sitting next to it gives time for the digestive juices to churn and prepare. The result? Better-digested food, less stress, less of a cortisol release and, therefore, a slimmer tummy. (Cortisol is a stress hormone that, in excess amounts, can lead to stubborn belly fat.) Even liquids (which I suggest you not drink with meals, since it dilutes digestive juices) should be mixed entirely with saliva before swallowing. Adhere to the old nutritional adage of "drink your foods and chew your liquids."

I realize it can be difficult to eat cleanly in such an unclean world. Nobody wants a reaction like the one seen in the commercial for a popular dating site, which shows a woman sitting with a date who is boring her with his dietary needs—"I am gluten-free, sugar-free, dairy-free," etc. She rolls her eyes and stands to leave, saying, "I'll call you when I'm 'free.'" But know that even though you may be the object of occasional ridicule, you will outlive many of your critics for making the clean food choices that you do.

Healthy Habit Helpers

1. Get a plan right now for what you will do the next time you want to eat fast food:

   _____

   _____

   _____

Now put your hand over your heart and pray this aloud with me:

God, I am ready for better health. I am willing to play my part in achieving it. Would You change my palate so that I enjoy the healthier foods I am going to try, and then grant me the discipline to maintain my new lifestyle? I know You will. I vow today to give this my best! In Jesus' name, Amen.

5

Get Your Beauty Sleep

How much sleep do you get each night? Chances are that your answer is "Not enough." I want to remind you of my testimony, which is that self-inflicted sleep deprivation almost killed me. God has miraculously designed your body to experience daily healing, but that happens once you enter deep, restorative sleep each night. The most important hours of your day happen when you are not even aware of them! Your body literally rejuvenates and renews. Now you know why Sleeping Beauty was so beautiful—she slept!

According to a *Huffington Post* article, "Your Body Does Incredible Things When You Aren't Awake," sleep deprivation can increase your risk of stroke, lead to obesity, increase diabetes risk, fuel memory loss, damage bones, increase cancer risk, hurt your heart and "kill you."[1]

But you never go to the doctor and receive a diagnosis of "sleep deprivation." Instead, it could be any of the resulting infirmities

1. Laura Schocker, "Your Body Does Incredible Things When You Aren't Awake," *Huffington Post*, March 10, 2014, http://www.huffingtonpost.com/20 14/03/07/your-body-does-incredible_n_4914577.html.

we just named, or fatigue, low libido, mental fogginess, mood swings, anxiety, weight gain, type 2 diabetes and more. And you know what? Those would all be legitimate diagnoses, and the prescription written would be a legitimate prescription for those legitimate problems. But neither addresses the root of the problem or the cure for it. The problem began with your sleep debt. The good news is that, with increased sleep and good nutrition, it can all be turned back around (worked for me). Without it, you will take the prescription, continue to sleep-deprive yourself and watch your body fall further and further apart, one illness at a time, until you die a needlessly early death.

In my 2014 book, *Seeing the Voice of God*, I set out to create a dreams book that fully explored the miracle of sleep itself, seeing as how sleep is the mattress of dreams! I interviewed a sleep-study doctor and gathered centuries of sleep data to help you get a better night's sleep and address any sleep disorders, and I even reviewed different sleep-study apps for your phone so that you could test yourself at home while you sleep. Of all the chapters in *Seeing the Voice of God*, I think I am most proud of those medical chapters because of the help they have provided for people to fall asleep, stay asleep and better remember their dreams, when they fortify their diets with the vitamins and minerals I suggest. I urge you to read it, but here I want to include from it an abbreviated version of my "Laura's ABCs for ZZZs Sleep Tips."[2] I am told by people all over the world that these tips are helping them sleep and dream again.

Laura's ABCs for ZZZs Sleep Tips

A. *Abstain from all caffeine (chocolate, soft drinks, nonherbal teas, diet pills, energy drinks, coffee), nicotine and alcohol,*

2. Laura Harris Smith, *Seeing the Voice of God: What God Is Telling You through Dreams and Visions* (Minneapolis: Chosen, 2014), 85–87.

since they can lead to insomnia. Alcohol may sometimes help you fall asleep, but you will not stay asleep, so for deep sleep, skip the nightcap. And smoking is not just bad for your lungs, but for sleep cycles due to waking up with nicotine withdrawals. Let this be the year that you rid your body of all such habit-forming, life-altering substances.

B. *Bedtime math.* Consider your required wake-up time the next morning and subtract at least 8½ hours from it to determine your bedtime. That allows 15 minutes to wind down (doing my sleep ABCs for ZZZs), 15 minutes to fall asleep and 8 hours to actually sleep. Aim to be at step C (below) 15 minutes before bedtime each night.

C. *Create room atmosphere and temperature.* As you are beginning your descent toward bedtime and heading to the bedroom or bathroom to prepare, use soft lighting to begin adjusting your circadian rhythms, which signals your brain to pump out the drowsy juice, melatonin. Adjust the temperature to a bit cooler and use a fan for white noise.

D. *De-stress for 5 minutes before climbing into bed.* Try a warm face wash, an Epsom salt bath (which is pure magnesium sulfate and aids sleep), essential oils on your pillow or any favorite relaxation routine to train your body that sleep is near. Be good to yourself and create your own bedtime traditions. Sleep time is a sacred time.

E. *Enter.* Time to transition into your bedclothes, bedroom and bed itself. Lie down, close your eyes and enter into peace. Ask God to enter your heart if you never have; then ask Him to enter your dreams and speak to you tonight.

F. *Forgive.* You have cleansed the atmosphere in your room; now cleanse the atmosphere of your heart. "Don't let the sun go down while you are still angry, for anger gives a foothold to the devil" (Ephesians 4:26–27 NLT). It is time to forgive whoever ruined your day or night, especially if it is the person lying next to you. What you go to bed with, you wake up with, so choose love. Ask God's forgiveness for whomever He brings to mind, and for yourself if necessary. Start fresh tomorrow.

G. *Go to sleep.* Find your "sweet spot" sleeping position. If you cannot fall asleep, try slowing down your breathing. This mirrors sleep stages N1 and N2[3]; you are basically tricking your brain into thinking you are there and causing your brain waves to slow down and widen (I have done this for years). If you still cannot fall asleep, try keeping a gratitude journal or reading, but use an actual book and not your tablet or phone, because the direct lights cue your pineal gland to quit making melatonin, the drowsy hormone. Pray Psalm 127:2 over yourself: "For so He gives His beloved sleep" (NKJV).

Too often we cannot sleep because of worry. If that describes you, I hope this poem helps you to rest—body, mind and spirit.

The Rest of God

Into a boat, and then out to sea
the disciples followed You toward Galilee

And they went, unsure of where they were going
They were just watching You—'til the wind started blowing

Then shifting their focus, and changing their gaze
their eyes were soon fixed on the wind and the waves

3. Ibid., 74–79.

Why is it perspective is so hard to keep?
And why, when I'm drowning, do You seem so asleep?

You slept in the boat as the waves formed great walls;
While they panicked, You dreamed and envisioned their
    calls

And the Sea of Galilee, with its undisturbed form
gave up its peace and gave way to storm

Its waters are shallow and still on all sides
Only twelve miles long, and a mere seven wide

So how do such waves form out of such peace
to record the worst storms in the whole Middle East?

With the great Mediterranean just fifty miles west
and Lebanon's mountains fifty northeast at best

The Sea of Galilee is nestled in between
and although it is usually still and serene

One low-pressure system coming from the Great Sea
crashes into those mountains, bouncing back on Galilee

And suddenly its waters are stirred and transformed
and from perfect peace comes a violent storm

O God, will it ever be different in me?
With these mountains I can't seem to cast to the sea?

Can You teach me to see them and not see their size?
Looking at them with faith and not with my eyes?

You're the God of all flesh, and that includes me
Can You speak to my mind like You spoke to the sea?

Since faith is the substance of those things not seen
I MUST walk by faith, not by sight, in between

And though storms rage near me, they will not within
I'll "be of good cheer" and choose joy to the end!

I will walk by my faith, I will walk on the sea;
I won't follow signs and wonders, but they'll follow me

And on that great day when my faith will be sight,
the faith of those watching will reach a new height

Calm my faith, calm my heart, Lord, calm the wind and
    waves, too
as I 'bide in this boat, full at rest next to You
© Laura Harris Smith

Healthy Habit Helpers

1. In the space below, do the bedtime math and determine what your regular nighttime routine needs to be to ensure better sleep and optimum health.

Now put your hand over your heart and pray this aloud with me:

Father, forgive my sleep rebellion, heal my sleep disorders and help me pay my sleep debt. I am Your beloved, and You give Your beloved sleep, so I receive Your rest. Amen.

6

Get Up and Scale Down

Face it. You love to be fit but hate fitness. Truth is, I prefer an exorcism to exercise. I mean, I can rebuke an unclean spirit from an individual and fully expect by faith that it is gone for good; so, then, why can I not just rebuke people's unclean diets for them? And why can I not rebuke calories for myself? The reason is because prayers for physical fitness are a lot like prayers for patience. The answer comes with our cooperation. So it is prayer *and* participation that gets the job done. I find that the way to keep my spiritual and physical flesh tamed and trimmed begins on my knees and is then carried out on my feet. Exorcise, then exercise!

I never remember my grandmother talking about exercise. Or "abs" or "glutes" or any other body part we obsess over today. She and my grandfather got a daily workout on their farm, along with their five children, one of whom was my mother. Same with my other grandparents and their twelve children, including my father. I wonder what that generation would think about the way we get our exercise today . . . standing still in one spot doing reps on a piece of exercise equipment. I am trying to imagine my grandparents' 1930s farmhouse even having a treadmill, elliptical stepper or weight bench. Absurd. There was no room in the house, and there was no electricity in the barn. Besides, they did **Exorcise, then exercise!** not need workout equipment because their workout involved actual work and left them dog tired by the end of each day. Jogging in place on a treadmill would have felt like "wasting time," and it *would* have been for them. Their bodies detoxed naturally through daily sweating, with the help of the hot south Georgia sun, and they mostly ingested food they grew themselves. I do not envy the hard farm life, but I do envy work being your workout. My work only leaves me with zero brain flab and strong fingers. After ten years of training, playing and competing in classical piano as a kid, I went straight to high school typing lessons and then on to the era of email and to writing books. A typing test today scored me at 110.35 words per minute with 100-percent accuracy. But in the words of my young grandson, Ezra, "Lollie, you're going to become a couch potato if you do not get up off this couch more." I asked him if he would like to finger wrestle, but he did not seem impressed.

So I have to be very intentional, not just about exercise but about . . . standing up. I am always on deadline, either with writing or editing or marketing, and even when I am doing radio or television, I am seated. During certain seasons I am sitting for sixteen hours daily, and then I am horizontal for the other eight—not conducive for a speedy metabolism. In my twenties, thirties and forties, when I was chasing six kids, I could eat whatever and not gain a pound, and now I see my three daughters enjoying that same season of womanhood. Now in my fifties, I have to remember that I am in the autumn of my life (ahem, late summer) and just be more deliberate with movement. My solution? I spent 160 dollars and bought a petite, foldaway treadmill that stays in my bedroom (and matches it); because I have to walk past it multiple times a day, I hop on and run a mile while I check social media, etc. Sometimes I get so consumed on my phone (just like you) that two or three miles have gone by without me knowing. Try it! (And, since you are wondering, it is the Confidence Power Plus Motorized Fitness Treadmill. You're welcome!)

Or consider trading in your desk chair for a large exercise ball (a.k.a. birthing ball). They are super easy to balance on, engage your "abs and glutes" just to stay upright, relieve tension as you lightly bounce while working or typing and are just plain fun. *Deskercise!*

No matter how challenging getting more exercise may feel, it is worth making a top priority. Did you know that diet and exercise determine obesity more than genetics? The *American Journal of Clinical Nutrition* published a study by Swedish scientists[1] who found that the fat mass and obesity–associated gene (the FTO gene, which has been linked to weight gain[2]) only increases your risk for obesity if you are also leading a sedentary lifestyle. So you are not shackled by your genes, but you do need to commit to moving. According to University of Oxford and Columbia University researchers, if today's obesity trends do not change, by the year 2030, 50 percent of the U.S. population will be obese, and there will be 7.8 million more diabetics, 6.8 million more people with coronary heart disease or strokes and 539,000 extra annual incidents of cancer.[3]

1. Emily Sonestedt, Charlotta Roos, Bo Gullberg, Ulrika Ericson, Elisabet Wirfält, and Marju Orho-Melander, "Fat and Carbohydrate Intake Modify the Association between Genetic Variation in the FTO Genotype and Obesity," *American Journal of Clinical Nutrition* 90, no. 5 (2009): 1418–1425, http://ajcn .nutrition.org/content/90/5/1418.full.

2. Louise Brunkwall, Ulrika Ericson, Sophie Hellstrand, Bo Gullberg, Marju Orho-Melander, and Emily Sonestedt, "Genetic Variation in the Fat Mass and Obesity-Associated Gene (FTO) in Association with Food Preferences in Healthy Adults," *Food and Nutrition Research* 57, no. 1 (2013), http://www.tandfonline .com/doi/full/10.3402/fnr.v57i0.20028.

3. Scott Christ, "Healthy Eating Statistics," *The Healthy Eating Guide* (blog), accessed April 21, 2017, http://www.thehealthyeatingguide.com/healthy-eating -statistics/.

You might wonder which weight/height scale I endorse—you know, the tables that calculate how much you should weigh based on your height. Actually, I don't. The trouble with them is that it puts the focus on a goal that is determined by the scale, which you could probably get to with some starvation or purging and be dangerously unhealthy at your ideal weight. Plus, it is frighteningly easy for the scales to become your god, meaning they are the fixation of your day in an idolatrous way. Instead, I say to focus on my "five to thrive" pillars of health and vitality:

1. A 75-percent vegetable and fruit diet
2. Drinking half your body weight in ounces daily, spread throughout the entire day (if you weigh 150 pounds, for example, then drink 75 ounces daily)
3. Resting eight hours each night
4. Daily exercise of some kind
5. Total endocrine hormonal balance: thyroid, adrenals (cortisol and adrenaline), pancreas (insulin), gonads (testosterone, estrogen, progesterone), etc.

You can wear all the baggy shirts, long necklaces, big scarves and slim wear you own to mask a growing waistline (trust me, I did it during one season), or you can just focus on these "five to thrive" pillars of vitality and watch your weight—and entire insides—take care of themselves!

Whatever you do, do not waste your time or money on low-fat or sugar-free foods. I am not saying to eat foods laden with bad fats and sugar, but you need to be educated so that you do not fall for the "low-fat" food trap—foods that, sure, may be low in bad fats but may also be too high in sodium and cholesterol. Let me take a moment to teach you how to read a food label so that you know what is really "living" inside your dead foods.

The nutrition facts label is placed by manufacturers on foods, medicinal teas, vitamins, supplements, etc. and is your glimpse into the nutrients within your nosh. Here are twenty things I bet you did not know your label does for you. Become familiar with them and shop smartly:

- DV is short for "daily values."
- Serving sizes are standardized to help consumers compare similar foods.
- Serving sizes use units like "cup" or "pieces."
- Serving sizes influence calories and nutrients listed at the top of the label.
- Using this, you can discover how many servings you are consuming.
- You can also determine caloric intake and nutrients provided.
- The calorie section of the label can help you manage your weight.
- Calories measure how much energy one serving provides.
- Fats, cholesterol and sodium content are listed first, since those are often overconsumed by Americans and need monitoring.
- Health experts suggest lowering intakes of trans fats, saturated fats and cholesterol.
- Look for products that are high in vitamin A, vitamin C, calcium, iron and dietary fiber.
- The footnote (with asterisk [*]) at the base of the label indicates that the "%DV" is based on a 2,000-calorie-a-day diet.
- The footnotes may be omitted if the label is too small.
- Use the %DV for total fat to quickly compare one food to another that claims to be "nonfat," "light" or "reduced fat."

- The three foods that do not have %DVs on the label are sugars, proteins and trans fats.
- If a product claims to be "high protein," then the label must list the %DV protein content.
- Sugars listed on a label include both natural and added sugars.
- Look for foods with little to no added sugars.
- These ten names for sugars can be found on labels: corn syrup, dextrose, sucrose, maltose, high fructose corn syrup, fruit juice concentrate, honey, maple syrup, evaporated cane juice and cane syrup.
- The ingredients list is found near the bottom of the label, and ingredients are listed according to their percentage of the whole, from largest to smallest.

In May 2016, the FDA announced that the nutrition facts label is changing, and food and beverage manufacturers were given until mid-2018 to comply with displaying the updated version on their products. FDA delays, however, have pushed back this deadline, with no definite compliance date cited, making it very difficult to know how to complete this healthy living habit for you (three drafts of it so far). I hope, before too long, we will all be benefiting from the new-and-improved labels. It should include these additions and more: "added sugars" must now be itemized, the font size has increased for "calories" and "serving sizes," and serving size measurements themselves have changed. You know how annoying it is to open a small snack and learn from the label that it counts as two servings (and, thus, you must double the calories)? Well, the new labels will reflect one serving, since people typically consume a small package in one sitting. You can find all the updates at the FDA's website.[4]

4. "Changes to the Nutrition Facts Label," U.S. Food and Drug Administration, updated April 25, 2017, accessed June 9, 2017, https://www.fda.gov/Food/Guid

Until then, you can still study the label-reading facts in this section, which will help you define the unchanging components of every nutrition fact label.

Today's prayer is in the form of a poem and follows your Healthy Habit Helper below.

Healthy Habit Helpers

1. Are you at your ideal weight? Write your basic health goals below in full:

_____

_____

_____

_____

_____

Now put your hand over your heart and pray this aloud with me:

I need to be more disciplined
I need a new routine
My flesh, though, is not interested
In what that just might mean

I'm quick to set a regimen
But slow at self-control
I wish there was a medicine
To help me meet my goal

anceRegulation/GuidanceDocumentsRegulatoryInformation/LabelingNutrition/ucm385663.htm.

If order's in my schedule, though
My flesh will learn the drill
And if I'll bridle whims and grow
My heart will train my will

Amen!

                  © *Laura Harris Smith*

7

Strike Oil

If I could point to the one thing we did as a family that changed the way we combat sickness, it would be prayer. I will talk more about that in our final healthy living habit, "Know Thy Healer." But if I had to name the number-one thing we did in the natural to *prevent* sickness, it would be incorporating essential oils into our lifestyle. They have been around since the third day of creation and are mentioned in the Bible 188 times—some claim as many as 600 times when you count the mentions of aromatic plants.

While it is quite impossible to tell you everything you need to know about essential oils in a few pages, we can get a good start! Chances are you have already used an essential oil before, even just for aromatherapy, but do you know what oils are best for stomachaches? What about for runny nose or jet lag or nausea? You will know by the end of this commentary!

I was first introduced to essential oils by my daughter Jessica, who had become a wellness advocate for a major essential oil distributor. She held an oil class one winter, and a certain kit was advertised as taking the place of every over-the-counter medicine in your medicine cabinet. I was intrigued. So I bought this basic kit, and because it cost more than a hundred dollars, it automatically signed me up as a wellness advocate, too. I did not tell anybody, and I basically just enjoyed the discount on our personal oils, but it was a decision that came in handy a few years later when I invented Quiet Brain® (my essential oil blend discussed in "De-stress Your Distress"). I knew oils well by then, where to get them and the pricing, making it easier for me to take the plunge into the oil business.

But I had nothing to teach me. I should have bought one of the countless essential oils books out there, but I honestly did not know of the vast subculture that surrounded oils at the time (and now it is not even "sub"). I did not care about which oils were good for balding or bunions. Just tell me what to do for a headache! I just needed the basics (what I am going to give you here, today), and so, with a little help from online testimonies and Google, I began experimenting on my king-sized family. It has now been four years since I have had to buy any pain relievers, abdominal treatments, first aid remedies or cold medicines.

Speaking of colds, let's talk prevention. The fact is that you do not "catch" a cold. You earn a cold. And I argue that a cold is not a cold at all, but a massive detox initiated when your system has had enough of processed foods and environmental toxins. True, viruses and germs are out there, but a healthy immune system should fight them all off. A cold results in considerable mucus production, which draws toxins providentially and **The fact is that you do not "catch" a cold. You earn a cold.** provides a means of exiting the body. Therefore, start looking at a cold as a detox that you have unfortunately earned through improper rest and poor nutrition. Improve both and be well. This theory also explains why no cure has been found for the common cold—and I am not the only health expert to subscribe to it.

So once the cold (detox) comes, what oils do you apply to relieve symptoms? First, let's define oil application methods, and then I will progress to a list of ailments and treatments. Because I do not know you, your doctor or your journey, I ask you to consult and consider all before adding any new treatments to your health regimen. It is always safer.

You can enjoy and employ essential oils in three main places: the body, the air and the water. Each has its own usage techniques:

The Body

Orally: Some essential oils can be taken by mouth, either with a few drops in a capsule or in a water tonic, 5 drops max. Check the bottle to see if any oil is safe to ingest.

Topically: Goes on the skin; either apply a max of 5 drops "neat" (directly on skin without dilution) or a max of 5 drops per teaspoon of carrier oil (olive, grape seed, almond, sesame, fractionated coconut, etc.). You can apply to pulse points (wrists), temples, neck, brainstem region (back of neck, just under hairline), bottoms of feet or directly on the region of discomfort (never in the eyes).

Nasally: Apply 2 drops on a tissue or handkerchief and place over nose (or under pillowcase at night) for deep breathing. Or hold bottle under nose and breathe deeply. The oil goes directly to the limbic areas of the brain through the nasal passages for rapid effect.

The Air

As when used nasally, essential oils are helpful and healthful when used in general aromatherapy. Try the following to liven up any space:

220

- Diffusers (activate oil and release it into air): 1–6 drops.
- Light bulbs: 1 drop on cool bulb. Smells once switched on.
- Fireplace wood: 3 drops per log (pine, cypress, cedarwood).
- Candles: 2 drops in candle once lit and heated. Avoid wick.
- Humidifiers: 2–8 drops directly in water. Refill and repeat.
- Spray bottles: 5 drops in warm water in bottle, then shake.

The Water

We all know our skin has a million little mouths on it, which is why what you soak in *seeps* in. Here are ideas for how to use oil with water:

- Bath: 8–10 drops after water is drawn. Soak and breathe.
- Epsom salt bath: 10 drops per cup of salts in warm water.
- Shower: 2 drops on scalp; 4 drops on cloth to scrub skin.
- Foot bath: 4–6 drops in hot water; soak 15 minutes.
- Spot bath: 3 drops in hot water; soak any area (e.g., hands).

And now, below is my "Famous Fifty Ouchie List": These are the fifty most common household ailments and which oils best support healing from them. You can choose whether you want to use them on the body, in the air or in water (or a combination of two or three for a greater effect). Remember that when applied topically you should never put oil in tender crevices; for example, for bladder/urinary tract infection, apply to the skin directly on top of the bladder and never internally. For stomach or constipation issues, avoid the rectum—but you can put oil drops in your navel or rub on the abdomen (or ingest by placing drops of oil in an empty gel capsule, if the bottle specifies that oral use is safe).

Acne: tea tree, lavender, lemongrass, frankincense, helichrysum

Allergies: peppermint, lemon, eucalyptus, basil, tea tree

Arthritis: frankincense, turmeric, wintergreen, peppermint, lavender, eucalyptus, ginger, rosemary, lemon

Athlete's foot: tea tree, lemon, peppermint, eucalyptus, lavender

Bites/stings: tea tree, lavender, basil

Bladder infection: lemongrass, oregano, clove, myrrh

Bronchitis/breathing: cinnamon, eucalyptus, peppermint, frankincense, ginger

Burns: Crack raw eggs on burn for immediate relief, then apply helichrysum, tea tree, lavender

Cold sores: lemon, lavender, frankincense, hyssop, tea tree

Cold symptoms: tea tree, rosemary, eucalyptus, oregano, clove

Constipation: ginger, fennel, sandalwood, black pepper, patchouli

Coughs: frankincense, eucalyptus, thyme, lavender, peppermint

Cuts: tea tree, lavender, eucalyptus, frankincense, myrrh, oregano

Detox: geranium, lemon, wild orange, grapefruit, oregano, ginger

Diaper rash: tea tree, lavender, chamomile

Diarrhea: peppermint, lavender, lemon, tea tree, orange, basil

Earache: Soak cotton ball in warm tea tree, basil, rosemary, lavender

Fever: Water-sponge body down with peppermint, lavender, eucalyptus

Fever blisters: Apply bergamot, lavender, tea tree, frankincense with Q-tip

Foot care: hyssop, lavender, frankincense

Gas: peppermint, dill, coriander, spearmint, eucalyptus

Halitosis (bad breath): lemon, lavender, spearmint, peppermint

Hay fever: chamomile, peppermint, lemon, lavender

Headache: wintergreen, frankincense, peppermint

Heartburn: eucalyptus, peppermint, lavender

Indigestion: peppermint, ginger, dill, coriander

Infertility: Female: cypress, geranium, thyme; Male: vetiver, basil

Insomnia: Quiet Brain contains the top eight brain-/mind-quieting oils

222

Jet lag: peppermint, grapefruit, eucalyptus

Leg cramps: geranium, cypress, lavender

Memory: rosemary, ginger, basil, black pepper

Menopause: clary sage, coriander, jasmine, geranium, lavender

Muscle pain: frankincense, wintergreen, lavender, marjoram, rosemary

Nail bed care: tea tree oil applied "neat" (no carrier oil) on nail bed

Nausea: fennel, lavender, coriander, peppermint

Pink eye/conjunctivitis: tea tree, lavender

PMS: grapefruit, Roman chamomile, clary sage, geranium, fennel, jasmine

Pneumonia: tea tree, eucalyptus, lemon, oregano, thyme

Rash: chamomile, lavender, lemon, sandalwood, juniper, rose

Runny nose: lemon, basil, eucalyptus, peppermint

Scalp care/dandruff: tea tree, lavender, rosemary, patchouli, thyme

Sinus issues: rosemary, peppermint, oregano, tea tree, basil, eucalyptus

Sore throat/laryngitis: Rub on throat or inhale steamed chamomile, thyme

Splinters: tea tree, lavender

Stomachache: fennel, peppermint, clove

Stress: Quiet Brain contains the top eight brain-/mind-quieting oils

Sunburn: Use spray bottle with aloe vera juice and peppermint, lavender

Toothache: clove, lemon, chamomile

Warts: cedarwood, cinnamon bark, clove, tea tree, lavender

Wrinkles: helichrysum, frankincense, lavender, Hawaiian sandalwood

As you can see from this list, certain oils have multiple uses and are worth keeping on hand at all times. Here are my top twelve "must have" essential oils:

chamomile   eucalyptus

cinnamon   frankincense

lavender	rosemary
lemon	tea tree (melaleuca)
oregano	wild orange
peppermint	wintergreen

(Note: You can find oil blends that combine some of these oils rather than buying them individually.)

Instead of antibiotics: Did you know that oil of oregano is nature's antibiotic, antiseptic and antifungal? You can put one drop in a bucket of water and mop your entire kitchen, so just imagine what it does to your insides! My six kids never once had to take antibiotics when they were growing up (which is amazing), and now that we have knowledge of what oil of oregano can do, it has become a "go-to" in all of our households. First sign of a bladder infection? Put 3–4 drops of oil of oregano in an empty gel capsule and take every 3–4 hours for 3–4 days. Feel a sore throat coming on? Same thing. The illness never fully manifests for us.

Instead of ibuprofen: Need an anti-inflammatory for headache, muscle pain or fever? Try frankincense! There is a good reason why the wise men brought Mary frankincense for her recovery. (And myrrh!) It has very potent infection-fighting antioxidants inside.

Instead of aspirin: Aspirin belongs to a class of compounds known as salicylates. Wintergreen is a plant that naturally contains methyl salicylate—in fact, its oil is almost 99 percent methyl salicylate. Amazing. This is why your bottle of wintergreen oil (if it is good medicinal grade) will come with a childproof cap. One 15-milliliter bottle of wintergreen oil is equivalent to about 85 adult aspirin tablets (3 drops of wintergreen equals one aspirin).

In closing, essential oils come from the leaves, flowers and resins of trees and plants. How marvelous and mysterious that you see a tree on the first page of Scripture in Genesis and on the last page in Revelation. Ask God to give you the wisdom to fathom what secrets His creation holds for your health.

> Along the bank of the river, on this side and that, will grow all kinds of trees used for food; their leaves will not wither, and their fruit will not fail. They will bear fruit every month, because their water flows from the sanctuary. Their fruit will be for food, and their leaves for medicine.
>
> Ezekiel 47:12 NKJV

Healthy Habit Helpers

No questions today, but take the time to shop online for some good medicinal-quality essential oils!

Now put your hand over your heart and pray this aloud with me:

God, You are amazingly creative in the medicines You give us. I desire to understand the wisdom in creation and how it can bring me health. Lead me to the right source and provision. Amen.

8

Quench Your Thirst

As I write this I am at 35,000 feet on a return flight from Denver, Colorado, where I have spent a glorious day with Dr. Marilyn Hickey and her daughter, Sarah Bowling. They both love the body, mind and spirit message as much as I do, and they have invited me a few times on their show, *Today with Marilyn and Sarah*, to chat about my various books. At age 86, Marilyn is showing no signs of slowing down and still travels to all continents doing healing crusades, preaching, having her books translated and more. Sarah is the director of Saving Moses, an international ministry that provides care to the children of human trafficking victims, so she is always in the air as well. Now that I have been around Marilyn several times, I have noticed something very consistent: She is always sipping on a bottle of water. Today when I got to her home, the first thing she did was offer me water. And this afternoon, upon arriving at Sarah's home, one of the first things *she* asked was, "You're drinking lots of water here, right?" You see, Denver is a high-altitude city that can easily dehydrate you if you are unaware or unaccustomed to it. On top of that, this was a day trip for me—I flew there and back in the same day, for a total of almost 2,300 air miles in less than sixteen hours, which can also lead to serious dehydration. (Plus my step-o-meter app tells me I walked 2.5 miles today in the airport, so my body needs extra hydration after that.) So here I sit in seat 2A, guzzling my water and praying I can convince you of the importance of hydration to your total body health.

If I had a dollar for every time someone told me they just cannot seem to remember to drink enough water every day, I would spend it buying all of them a bottle of water! Please. You remember to eat. You remember to sleep. You listen to your body when it needs to go to the bathroom. Can you seriously not just get a hydration plan for your life? I hope what I have to say will persuade you to try. Again.

Ellen G. White (1827–1915) was a Christian pioneer and author of more than forty books and five thousand periodical articles that were translated into more than 160 languages, making her the most translated American author of all time. She also recorded more then two thousand dreams and visions, through which God deposited nuggets of wisdom in her concerning the body, mind and spirit. Fascinating! *Counsels on Diet and Foods* (Review and Herald Publishing Association, 1938) was published after her death and contained these nuggets from excerpts of the more than one hundred thousand pages she was estimated to have written while on earth. In it she writes of water:

> "Water is one of heaven's choicest blessings. Its proper use promotes health. It is the beverage which God provided to quench the thirst of animals and man." ~Ellen G. White

Water is one of heaven's choicest blessings. Its proper use promotes health. It is the beverage which God provided to quench the thirst of animals and man. Drunk freely, it helps to supply the necessities of the system, and assists nature to resist disease. Thousands have died for want of pure water and pure air who might have lived.[1]

Here are some friendly tips I can offer you for what works to remind me to hydrate:

1. **Keep water nearby.** I have a glass of filtered water near me at all times, a big mason jar that I fill up several times a day. Water is on the nightstand when I sleep, the end table when I write and stashed in my purse when I am on the run.

2. **Set phone reminders or alarms.** I have a reminder that goes off on my phone every two hours to remind me to hydrate. I have programmed in little quips like "Time for your afternoon guzzle!" or "Chug-a-lug, Laura!" I do the same to remind me to take my vitamins and for exercise. And then, yes, I also have one that says, "Laura, GO TO BED!" I have these on the computer, too, so quite often I get them in stereo. Just a little buzz, but it gets my attention so I can read the command and comply. You might think it is crazy, but if your excuse is that you are too busy, then why not take advantage of a little technological help? Besides, *it works*! (Aaaaand I kid you not, my evening "Time to guzzle water, Laura!" reminder just went off. The lady in 2C did not mind a bit; turns out she is a doctor. So drink up—doctor's orders!)

3. **Find your favorite water recipe.** *"Recipe?"* Yes. If you cannot seem to get excited about H_2O, then liven it up a bit. Try a SodaStream machine that makes carbonated water and then squeeze in some lime or lemon (my fave). I just refill the same mason jar all day long, and by day's end it

---

1. Ellen G. White, *Counsels on Diet and Foods* (Washington, D.C.: Review and Herald Publishing Association, 1938), 419.

contains so many lemon wedges that it hardly has room for water. But vitamin C is a great detoxifier! Lemons are high in antioxidants, which slow aging. Want proof? You know that trick you use to keep a peeled banana or apple from browning by squirting some lemon juice on it? Well, the brown means that the fruit is "dying." That is the process of oxidation, and every living thing goes through it. But lemon juice is an *anti*oxidant, so when it comes in contact with the peeled fruit, it preserves it. Just imagine what sipping lemon water does to slow down the aging process of your insides! Stop right now and go make some! I will include my own Fountain of Youth Detox Water recipe at the end of this commentary.

4. **Mark a gallon jug.** Google the words *gallon jug water marks* and get inspired at the pictures! Although you probably will not be drinking a gallon of water each day (although I know people who do), you can take a magic marker to that jug (or a one- or two- liter bottle) and create little phrases and water line reminders to mark your progress (basically serving the same purpose as the phone or computer reminders). Smart! Just find a plan that works for you.

5. **Find your quota.** As a simple rule, drink in ounces half of your body weight in pounds (120 pounds body weight = 60 ounces of water daily). Spread it out throughout the day so that you are not diluting your stomach acids, which are vital for digestion.

6. **Buy a water filtration system.** Back when I was first re-thinking my kitchen and replacing microwaves with a convection toaster oven, bottled juices with a juicer, table salt with pink salt, etc., buying a water filtration system seemed light-years away. I knew we needed it, because today's tap water is filled with chlorine and other harsh

chemicals. Then I found a great one from Aquasana for around 150 dollars, and my husband and I gave it to each other for Christmas. I highly recommend it, and your body will thank you forever! Filtered water pitchers are a start, but neither they nor your refrigerator's water filter can remove all the toxins from your drinking water. You need one that will not only cleanse it of chemicals but also other people's medications that have gone down into the sewage systems, into your local river and then back up into your faucets (after a good dose of added chlorine). I hate to be graphic, but now you know! Invest in an under-counter water filtration system.

Fountain of Youth Detox Water

1 cucumber, thinly sliced

1 lemon, sliced

1 orange, sliced

10 mint leaves

Add to one pitcher filtered water and let sit overnight

Two-thirds of your body is composed of water. Interestingly, roughly two-thirds of the earth's surface is also composed of water. Physically healthy people hydrate often. Get a plan today for how you will better steward this gift God has given you: water.

Healthy Habit Helpers

1. Get a hydration strategy today! Jot down ideas you have here:

_____

_____

_____

_____

Now put your hand over your heart and pray this aloud with me:

God, thank You for water. So many do not have it. Help me to get a plan and to have the discipline to keep my body's thirst quenched. Amen.

9

Live Life in the Fast Lane

This healthy living habit is probably not about what you are thinking it is. Unless, of course, you were hoping for something that will help you go deeper with God, hear His voice with crystal clarity and tear down demonic strongholds that may have been hindering your life. Surprise! This is a discussion about fasting.

I did not fast at all until I was 29 years old. Somehow, I did not even see the biblical principle in Scripture. I never even knew a single, solitary person who had fasted, and I was raised in church and was around very godly Christians every day of those 29 years. But I blame no one but myself. I had read the Bible through countless times by that age, and so I had obviously read the passages on fasting (over and over). Jesus said in Matthew 6:16, "*When* you fast," not, "*If* you fast." Why did I think His words did not apply to me? Sadly, they were not illuminated until I got around people who had lifestyles of fasting prayer; but once the illumination came, I stepped into a whole new world.

Do you have a door that you *know* you are supposed to walk through but it will not open? Fast. Do you have a sin issue in your life that you cannot seem to shake? Fast. Do you have a relationship that seems to be under constant siege or an infirmity that you need healing from? Fast, fast, fast! In my decades of walking with God, I have never discovered any other discipline that brings such great and immediate return as fasting. Demons must cower and angels must rush in at the hint of a praying saint. When I fast, I feel my spiritual ears open and my heart become more alert. I feel my spiritual feet pointing in the right direction toward whatever big decision I am facing, and it seems like a red carpet just rolls right out in front of me. All of my books are written with a food fast built in, including this one. You would think you could not write without proper brain fuel, and while that is normally true when I am not fasting (just "hungry"), on a fast there seems to be a special turbo-grace for endless inspiration.

My very first fast was a real doozy. It was spring of 1994, and a friend and I decided to embark upon a 21-day fast together. We were giddy with excitement. We wanted to do a fast of only water and no food at all. We decided to include sackcloth and ashes, so at night we would pray (individually in our homes), apply ashes to our foreheads and sleep in burlap sackcloth. (Our husbands were real sports!) We decided to wear no makeup, which, if you know me, you know is a big deal. Lo and behold, I forgot that I had to renew my license during this time, and so the glorious picture followed me around for five years! I had heard the Lord say I could have three things during the fast: water, mineral oil and chewing gum. I was quite puzzled at that directive. What was mineral oil, and why would I want it? And surely chewing gum was cheating. I thought for certain I had not heard God correctly, so I asked one of my church leaders. He told me the mineral oil would help lubricate my digestive system to prevent discomfort and that chewing gum was a must if I wanted to keep my friends, since fasting breath can be lethal. It encouraged me

> Do you have a relationship that seems to be under constant siege or an infirmity that you need healing from? Fast, fast, fast!

greatly that God would care about the minutiae of this fast, and those 21 days catapulted me into an entirely new spiritual realm (though I still laugh at the sackcloth part).

Since then, I have "enjoyed" many fasts, and I would like to share some helpful tips with you.

To start off, let's take a look at various lengths of fasts. There is an old fasting adage that says, "The longer the fast, the stronger the fast." I can vouch for that, but I encourage you to start where you can and build your fasting muscles over time. Here are the fasting lengths we see in Scripture:

1. Short (one- or two-meal) fasts—Genesis 24:32–33; 2 Samuel 1:11–12
2. One-day fasts—Ezra 9:5; Judges 20:26; 1 Samuel 7:5–6; 20:34
3. Three-day fasts—Esther 4:15–16; Acts 9:8–9
4. Seven-day fasts—1 Samuel 31:11–13; 2 Samuel 12:16, 18
5. Twenty-one-day fasts—Daniel 10:2–3
6. Forty-day fasts—Exodus 34:28; 1 Kings 19:8; Luke 4:1–2
7. Fasts of unspecified length—1 Samuel 1:7; 1 Kings 13:8–9; 21:27

Now you know the biblical fasting lengths—but keep in mind that the Lord will sometimes call you to fast for another period of time (like during a five-day conference you are attending, etc.). Let's look now at fasting types:

Normal fast: abstaining from food for a certain amount of time, ingesting only water or juices

Partial fast: limited eating (e.g., eating one meal a day) or a restricted diet all day long

Absolute fast: abstaining from food *and* liquids for a short duration (such as the three-day fast that Esther called)

Ration fast: eating or omitting certain food groups like breads or only eating fruits and vegetables

Activity fast: abstaining from a favorite activity or interest

Now I want to guide you through some biblical fasting models. About twenty years ago I was introduced to Elmer L. Towns's teachings on fasting that came from his book *Fasting for Spiritual Breakthrough*,[1] and I highly recommend you read it. Dr. Towns outlines nine fasting models, which I will only name for you here and leave it to you to purchase his book and learn what each one entails. I have also added one of my own at the end (the Hannah fast).

The disciple's fast, for breaking addiction: to loose the bands of wickedness (Isaiah 58:6), freeing ourselves and others from addiction to sin.

The Ezra fast, for solving problems: to undo heavy burdens (Isaiah 58:6); to solve problems, inviting the Holy Spirit's help in lifting our loads and overcoming barriers that keep ourselves and our loved ones from walking in the joy of the Lord.

The Samuel fast, for winning people to Christ: to let the oppressed go free (Isaiah 58:6) for revival and soul winning; to identify with people everywhere enslaved literally or by sin and praying to be used of God to bring people out of the kingdom of darkness into the light of God.

The Elijah fast, for emotional problems: to break the yoke (Isaiah 58:6), conquering the mental and emotional problems that would control our lives and returning the control to the Lord.

1. Elmer L. Towns, *Fasting for Spiritual Breakthrough: A Guide to Nine Biblical Fasts* (Minneapolis: Bethany House, 2017), 5–6.

The widow's fast, for humanitarian needs: to share our bread with the hungry and to care for the poor (Isaiah 58:7); to meet the needs of others.

The Saint Paul fast, for insight and decision making: to allow God's light to break forth like the morning (Isaiah 58:8), bringing clearer perspective and insight as we make critical decisions.

The Daniel fast, for health and physical healing: so our health shall spring forth (Isaiah 58:8), for gaining a healthier life or for healing.

The John the Baptist fast, for an influential testimony: that our righteousness shall go before us (Isaiah 58:8), that our testimonies and influence for Jesus will be enhanced before others.

The Esther fast, for protection from the evil one: that the glory of God will protect us from the enemy (Isaiah 58:8).

The Hannah fast, for a child or children to be born: to resist our rival, who would provoke us to believe that children are not possible for us (1 Samuel 1:7).

So now all you must do is choose the length, style and biblical model for your fast, and you are set! If you would like an additional fasting resource, feel free to go to my website's online store and download my free fasting e-book, *Hunger For God.*[2]

Healthy Habit Helpers

1. Do you have a regular lifestyle of fasting? I suggest at least one fast per quarter or more, of whatever length God leads. When could you begin a fast?

2. Laura Harris Smith, *Hunger For God,* 2nd ed., 2016, http://www.Laura HarrisSmith.com/store.html.

_____

_____

Now, put your hand over your heart and pray this aloud with me:

Jesus, I know You set the example for us of fasting. I ask for Your strength, discipline and revelation as I vow to make fasting a greater part of my walk with You. In Your name I pray, Amen.

10

Know Thy Healer

I need to be in health, Lord
This road has been so long
It's been a good few years, God
But today, I'm not so strong

It was another hard one
My head wants to explode
Along with my broad shoulders
It carries quite a load

My health is in Your hands, God
I have great peace of mind
But in this unhealed body
That peace remains confined
                    © Laura Harris Smith

I used to not believe in healing. I believed more in God's grace to endure sickness, which does occasionally come in handy; but to be the child of a miracle-working, death-defying, sea-parting, way-making God and yet never ask Him to work a miracle is just plain silly. And selfish. *And* a poor use of resources. God needs to be "allowed" and *invited* to be fully God. You may not be comfortable with the idea of being able to limit God's power, but Matthew 13:58 (NIV) tells us that Jesus "did not do many miracles [in Nazareth] because of their lack of faith."

Imagine having the power to limit Jesus. Well, you do. Imagine now the endless possibilities when you do not limit Him.

As we have said many times in this book, as the Trinity, God is three parts; and we, made in His image, are also three parts. As a result, He goes against His very being unless He offers healing to all three: body, mind and spirit. But when I began discovering healing Scriptures for the first time, I became overwhelmed—not only because I was ashamed at not having known there were more than a thousand healing Scriptures from Genesis to Revelation, but because I knew I needed to categorize them so I could be prepared to use them. When sickness comes, it is almost too late, because you are so focused on managing symptoms. For this very reason I created my "Ten Healing Commandments."[1] They first appeared in *The 30-Day Faith Detox*, but I am revisiting them here with an upgrade. As before, each commandment stands alongside its scriptural basis, but now it also comes with a follow-up question and a bit of homework. I am providing some space for you to answer directly in this book, because I want these next few pages to become an altar for you. I want your heart (and body) to kneel here and then stand up changed. If any unbelief in your soul is preventing God from doing a miracle for you, you are about to confront it. If any impatience in your heart is preventing Him from healing you by process, you are about to confront that, too. So read each healing commandment out loud, then its Scripture, and move on to the question, recording your answer in the space provided.

1. Smith, *Faith Detox*, 137–139.

1. **I am the Lord, thy Healer, and thou shalt have no other healers before Me.** Exodus 15:26: "For I am the LORD, your healer."

   Homework: Name all the healers in your life (medicines, remedies, nutritionists, doctors, etc.). This is not to discount them, but to help you prioritize God as the primary Healer. Take a moment and list what or whom you reach for first when sick (instead of prayer). Focus in the future on seeking God first for healing or a healing strategy, should sickness come.

   _____

   _____

2. **Thou shalt receive My healing Scriptures.** Psalm 107:20: "He sent out his word and healed them, and delivered them from their destruction."

   Homework: Name one healing Scripture you have a hard time believing or understanding. Consider how this confusion prevents you from receiving it as God's promise in your life. Confront it prayerfully and deal with it today.

   _____

   _____

3. **Thou shalt not be offended at healings or miracles.** Matthew 11:5–6 (and Luke 7:22–23): "The blind receive their sight and the lame walk, lepers are cleansed and the deaf hear, and the dead are raised up, and the poor have good news preached to them. And blessed is the one who is not offended by me."

Homework: Name a time when someone told you he or she was healed and you experienced doubt or offense. Maybe you felt awkward discussing it because something in your heart had trouble reconciling that person's healing with all the other healings you have not seen come to pass. Really think through (in writing) this emotional process and how you can be better prepared to filter testimonies you hear through God's Word and come out stronger in faith.

4. **Thou shalt live righteously in gratitude for My Son's stripes.** 1 Peter 2:24 (KJV): "Who his own self bare our sins in his own body on the tree, that we, being dead to sins, should live unto righteousness: by whose stripes ye were healed."

   Homework: Name any area where you are not "living righteously" (not living in right standing with God), thereby appearing to God to be ungrateful for Jesus' sacrifice for your every sin and sickness.

5. **Thou shalt not fear sickness.** Jeremiah 30:12, 17 (NKJV): "For thus says the LORD: 'Your affliction is incurable, your wound is severe. There is no one to plead your cause, that you may be bound up; you have no healing medicines. . . . I will restore health to you and heal you of your wounds,' says the LORD."

Homework: What is the first thing you do when you feel a sickness coming on, or when you receive a diagnosis from a helpful doctor? (For example, feel fear that you are about to miss work, fill a prescription, broadcast your diagnosis, begin declaring healing over your situation in prayer, etc.) What should you do to better position yourself to receive from the Lord?

_____

_____

6. **Thou shalt take care of thy body.** 1 Corinthians 3:16: "Do you not know that you are God's temple and that God's Spirit dwells in you?"

   Homework: Name a few ways that you take poor care of your body, or ways in which you can improve. If you are brave, document your weight and goals for the future.

   _____

   _____

7. **Thou shalt eat thy fruits and vegetables.** Genesis 1:29: "And God said, 'Behold, I have given you every plant yielding seed that is on the face of all the earth, and every tree with seed in its fruit. You shall have them for food.'"

   Homework: Is your diet 75 percent fruits and vegetables, as it should be? List those new vegetables and fruits you are going to add to your diet, and list those foods you are going to start omitting for better overall health.

   _____

   _____

8. **Thou shalt ask for the anointing oil.** James 5:14–15: "Is anyone among you sick? Let him call for the elders of the church, and let them pray over him, anointing him with oil in the name of the Lord. And the prayer of faith will save the one who is sick, and the Lord will raise him up. And if he has committed sins, he will be forgiven."

Homework: Name the last time you were anointed with oil. How do you feel about anointing oil? Why is it important to ask for it versus just being anointed without your permission?

_____

_____

9. **Thou shalt believe.** Matthew 13:58: "And he did not do many mighty works there, because of their unbelief."

Homework: This is your final opportunity to deal with any unbelief concerning miracles or healings. We live in a doubtful world and must always remind ourselves to choose faith. Take one more look into your heart and ask God to show you any place that trusts man more than Him.

_____

_____

10. **Thou shalt lay hands on the sick.** Mark 16:17–18: "And these signs will accompany those who believe: in my name they will cast out demons; they will speak in new tongues; they will pick up serpents with their hands; and if they drink any deadly poison, it will not hurt them; they will lay their hands on the sick, and they will recover."

Homework: Going beyond receiving healing means to give it away. Have you ever laid your hands on someone else and asked God to heal that person? What happened? Have you ever prayed for someone and seen him or her made well (physically, emotionally or spiritually)? List those experiences here, then continue making yourself available to God to be used as His agent to bring healing to others. Who do you know that needs healing right now?

_____

_____

Let the Scriptures convince you of His healing power for your spirit, mind and body. He wants you to ask for healing, just like you once asked for salvation, and He wants you to take yes for an answer. But you also must make wise nutritional choices so you can walk in divine health. It is staying smart so that you need less crisis intervention.

For more than twenty years, we have had a sign hanging inside our medicine cabinet that says, "DO NOT ingest any medicine from this cabinet unless you have first prayed for and ingested the healing Word of God." And then it states that believers will lay hands on the sick and they will recover (Mark 16:17–18), and that the prayer of faith will make the sick person well (James 5:14–15). This sign went up in the early 1990s, when we first gained revelation that Christ was our Healer, because we figured it was only natural to talk to Him in times of sickness. Instead of immediately reaching for the boxed meds or the phone to call the doctor, we simply pray first. Sometimes we were definitely prompted to call the doctor after prayer. Other times, we just knew it was going to be supernaturally taken care of—and every one of those times, it was. I would never tell anyone to make the same decisions we did, nor am I

244

antidoctor. (In fact, I am in nutrition school once again working toward my degree as a doctor of naturopathy.) But the point is, we made those decisions, and now our children know how to make them. Today, all of my adult children know their Healer. They know where He is and what He does. They know how to access healing, but they also understand their role in stewarding divine health. They are aware. The sign has faded in that medicine cabinet, and the "medicine" is all different now, too: only oils, vitamins, tonics and tinctures. But the Healer remains the same. And He is in it all.

Now put your hand over your heart and pray this aloud with me:

God, You *are my primary care Physician. Amen.*

OUTRO

A Photo Finish

Ever heard of a photo finish? It is when multiple contestants in a race finish at what appears to be the very same time, requiring a photograph to see who exactly came across the finish line first. My prayer is that as you enjoyed this book, your body, mind and spirit were in a race toward better health and that it will be a photo finish with three equal winners. That is the only way *you* will be the winner. *That* is the only path toward wholeness.

Let's take a moment and review everything you just learned. I enjoyed coming up with creative titles for these healthy living habits, like "Get the Word Out," "Bury the Hatchet" and "Don't Eat and Run!" But if you boil down the titles, they become straightforward directives. First, let's recap your top 10 spiritual directives:

1. Believe in miracles.
2. Pray in the Spirit.
3. Experience Spirit baptism.
4. Read your Bible *daily*.

5. Honor authority.
6. Attend church weekly (at least).
7. Guard your salvation.
8. Let Christ be your "go-to."
9. Choose faith and dodge doubt.
10. Be sure you are saved.

Next, your top 10 emotional directives:

1. Organize your environment.
2. Organize your time and flow.
3. Be courteous to others.
4. Smile more.
5. Laugh a lot!
6. Avoid stress.
7. Refuse discouragement.
8. Know when to withdraw (go where you can submit).
9. Choose your friends (and spouse) wisely.
10. Forgive more.

And, finally, your top 10 physical directives:

1. Improve your nutrition.
2. Eat your vegetables and fruits.
3. Limit meat, wheat and sweets.
4. Avoid fast food and eating food fast.
5. Sleep eight hours each night.
6. Exercise and watch your weight.
7. Use essential oils.
8. Drink half your body weight in ounces, daily.

9. Develop a fasting lifestyle.

10. Receive God's healing power.

Congratulations! Behold the new you! Refer back to your handwritten notes at the end of each commentary to remind you to stay on track.

And now some final advice on how to handle the naysayers you may encounter as you begin implementing your new healthy living habits. You are about to emerge as a new-and-improved you, and people are going to take notice, even as you first make the smallest of alterations. This is going to bring conviction to a great number of people around you and lead to some interesting conversations, leaving you feeling like the teacher you did not want to be in certain relationships. But you will be ready because it is personal revelation to you, and no one can deny a testimony. For example, your friend finishes giving the waitress his unhealthy double cheeseburger with chili fries and a cola order, and now it is your turn. You order your megasalad with lean chicken, olive oil with lemon wedges for dressing and bottled water with a lemon slice to drink. Like a rising Pig-Pen dust cloud, you can feel the guilt emanating from your convicted friend. The waitress takes the menus and leaves, and suddenly there is an awkward moment in which your friend feels led to defend his selection, or he admits he needs change and says he admires your fortitude. Either way, here is your open door. The words you say could possibly add ten years to your friend's life if he follows through. Share with him *why* you are on the journey you are, and encourage him to begin his own. You are now an authority! Maybe recommend *The Healthy Living Handbook*.

Occasionally (not often), someone will misunderstand my body, mind and spirit message as being a "works" doctrine. It is usually someone from the Spirit-filled community, of which I am a card-carrying charismatic clergy member, so I know how "we" think and therefore am qualified to say what I am about to say. At first glance, these people think I am undermining the supernatural realm with my natural remedies. You might encounter the same misconceptions. Some think a dramatic deathbed healing is more newsworthy than a lifetime of no sickness at all. Many of these are the ones with the works doctrine, because *it takes a lot of work to get chronically sick*. It does not happen overnight. And if overeating earned them those chronic illnesses, it was not the devil who handed them out. It *was* the devil who tempted them to overeat, but they yielded to him. So is it really right to beg God for a miracle when we have no plans to change our sinful lack of self-control that welcomed the infirmity? God will often still heal, but blessed is the man who maintains his miracle. Could this perhaps be the answer to the question, "Why does God heal some and not others?" Maybe He heals all. Maybe few maintain it. *However*, if you have lost a loved one to an infirmity after he or she had a lifelong history of a healthy lifestyle, then I submit to you that it was just your loved one's time to meet the Lord. I am speaking more about those people who eat from hell's kitchen and expect heaven to bless it. And some people adopt a

God will often still heal, but blessed is the man who maintains his miracle. healthy lifestyle late in life but perhaps are unable to reverse damage they have already imposed upon themselves, or perhaps they did not understand how to intercede and break the generational curses in their family's medical history and so they were not healed. Please take my comments in context and know that my goal is to promote a lifestyle of participation with God to achieve the divine health you are praying for.

I have been "talked down to" at ministers' gatherings by people who believed God made all the foods and that they should be able to enjoy them. (If only we still had the exact foods God made, but, alas, there are no heritage seeds on the earth, and we can say with great certainty that God did not make the gluttonous gluten in today's wheat.) It was as if my message somehow contradicted faith and miracles. One of them had even been recently diagnosed with cancer (which was surgically removed) and yet planned no dietary changes. That person admitted trying to make dietary changes at first but said it felt like bondage, deciding to "choose faith" instead—and hinting that my life's work required no faith or was less miraculous. So I entreat you . . .

Consider the pear. It fights off free radicals, protects against heart disease and high cholesterol, controls diabetes and prevents cancer. Pears are so wholesome, hypoallergenic and safe that they are usually one of the first foods given to infants. With all that power-packed purity, are pears really any less miraculous than prayers?

The "one and done" prayer camp need not worry about Laura Harris Smith's motives or faith for instant miracles. Remember that Healthy Living Habit No. 1 included the testimonies of the first miracles I ever saw while praying over people: the one man whose leg grew right into my hands and the other man healed of HIV. But healing works exactly the same as salvation. I like getting people saved and forgiven of their sins, but I also like them to quit sinning. Likewise, I like getting people miraculously healed, but I also like to help them stay healed and walk in divine health.

I do pray that you now feel the discipline of divine health is within your grasp. If so, I have done my job. If you will now do yours, I proclaim you will make the world a better place, starting with your own and the people in it whom you have been called to influence. Amen!

"The world is at long last experiencing the bracing reality check that they cannot fix their weight problems with a fad diet, their emotional problems with a better relationship or their spiritual problems without a healthy faith," says Laura Harris Smith. "People have tried unsuccessfully for several generations now to 'fix themselves' with one nonbiblical fad after another by segregating their whole being and focusing on either the body, mind or spirit. You can feel the collective shrug of society's shoulders as they are conceding that wholeness only comes God's way, by addressing all three."

Laura is a certified nutritional counselor and has a bachelor's degree in original medicine. She is the author of multiple books, including the bestsellers *The 30-Day Faith Detox: Renew Your Mind, Cleanse Your Body, Heal Your Spirit* (Chosen Books, 2016) and *Seeing the Voice of God: What God Is Telling You through Dreams and Visions* (Chosen Books, 2014). She is also continuing her body, mind and spirit education by pursuing her doctorate in original medicine.

"Good bodily nutrition leads first to healthier days and more restful nights," teaches Laura, "then to improved dream recall and better communication with God, all of which results in thriving spiritual and emotional health. Who wouldn't want all that? I live to motivate and educate people to possess it."

Laura speaks and ministers across denominational lines and is known for bringing a lighthearted look at the heaviest of biblical topics. Married for 33 years, Laura and her husband,

Chris, have six children—Jessica, Julian, Jhason, Jeorgi, Jude and Jenesis—and reside near Nashville, Tennessee. With half of the kids now grown and married, the "grandmuffins" now outnumber the kids.

Invite Laura to speak at booking@LauraHarrisSmith.com.

Official website: LauraHarrisSmith.com

Make sure to take advantage of Laura's *Healthy Living Handbook* videos at her YouTube site: www.YouTube.com /LauraHarrisSmith

See the videos as they are released live by liking Laura's Facebook author page: Facebook.com/LauraHarrisSmithPage

Twitter: @LauraHSmith

Chris and Laura's Nashville church: EastgateCCF.com